MODERN TECHNIQUES
OF
VOCAL REHABILITATION

Publication Number 849
AMERICAN LECTURE SERIES®

A Monograph in
The BANNERSTONE DIVISION *of*
AMERICAN LECTURES IN SPEECH AND HEARING

Edited by
CHARLES F. DIEHL

Speech and Hearing Center
Department of Special Education
College of Education
University of Kentucky
Lexington, Kentucky

Second Printing

MODERN TECHNIQUES

OF

VOCAL REHABILITATION

By

MORTON COOPER, Ph.D.

Formerly Director, Voice and Speech Pathology, Outpatient Clinic
Clinical Assistant Professor
Head and Neck Surgery Division
UCLA Center for the Health Sciences
Los Angeles, California
Presently in Private Practice
Los Angeles, California

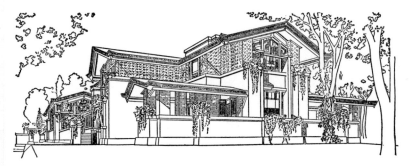

CHARLES C THOMAS · PUBLISHER
Springfield · Illinois · U.S.A.

Published and Distributed Throughout the World by
CHARLES C THOMAS • PUBLISHER
BANNERSTONE HOUSE
301-327 East Lawrence Avenue, Springfield, Illinois, U.S.A.

© *1973, by* CHARLES C THOMAS • PUBLISHER
ISBN 0-398-02451-0
Library of Congress Catalog Card Number: 72-75913

First Printing 1973
Second Printing 1974

Printed in the United States of America
N-1

To

my wife, Marcia Ann Hartung Cooper,
without whom this book could not have been written
and to my daughters
Lorna and Marla

FOREWORD

This is a highly personal book in which the author offers a practical guide to voice therapy based on his extensive clinical experience. Although a traditionalist by training he deviates sufficiently from classical approaches to be both unique and controversial. His innovative techniques, shifts of emphasis in therapy, and occasional disagreement with acknowledged authorities will disturb some and please others; but, whatever the reaction, his therapeutic results are impressive enough to command the attention of his colleagues and all others interested in the management of vocal disorders.

HENRY J. RUBIN, M.D.
Senior Attending, Department of
Otolaryngology, Cedars-Sinai Medical Center,
Los Angeles; Associate Clinical Professor,
University of California at Los Angeles
School of Medicine

PREFACE

Modern Techniques of Vocal Rehabilitation emphasizes simplified, specific techniques to alleviate and/or eliminate all types of functional and organic dysphonias. Essentially, the material is based on this author's clinical experience as a private practitioner and as former director and therapist of the Voice and Speech Clinic, Head and Neck Surgery Division, UCLA School of Medicine. The text outlines the problems confronting the voice therapist in schools, in clinics, and in private practice and emphasizes the important aspects that must be understood by the therapist in order to achieve successful vocal rehabilitation.

This material is also intended to provide background information for professionals in allied fields seeking an overview of vocal rehabilitation. It will be of assistance to physicians, psychiatrists, psychologists, speech teachers, dentists, orthodontists, and, in general, to anyone interested in understanding the process of vocal rehabilitation, the symptomatology of voice disorders, the methods for correcting defective voices, and the problems inherent in overcoming a voice disorder.

To Friedrich S. Brodnitz, M.D., I wish to express gratitude for guiding me into the field of vocal rehabilitation.

Professional associates of past and of present to whom I am indebted for their patience and presence include: Virgil Anderson, Ph.D., Elise Hahn, Ph.D., John Snidecor, Ph.D., Lee Edward Travis, Ph.D., the late Robert West, Ph.D., and the late Joel J. Pressman, M.D.

I wish to thank the laryngologists and other physicians who have given me the opportunity to be of assistance to them and to their patients.

I also wish to thank my patients for placing their trust in modern techniques of vocal rehabilitation.

To Virginia Agnello, M.A., my deep appreciation for her assistance in preparing the manuscript for publication.

A final point of acknowledgement is to Marcia Ann Hartung Cooper, M.A., my wife and collaborator, for her continued prodding and constant support in the writing and completion of this book.

MORTON COOPER

INTRODUCTION

This book is written from extensive clinical experience with voice cases, supported with numerous before and after tapings of patients, and confirmed, when possible, by follow-up investigations, all of which assist in defining the progress or lack of progress in therapy for patients. The material presented is practical, not theoretical.

The vast majority of all voice disorders were found to have been caused or perpetuated by use of either an incorrect pitch level, more often too low than too high, or an improper tone focus, which usually emphasizes laryngopharyngeal resonance.

The location and maintenance of the optimal or natural pitch and the proper tone focus for the voice patient are of primary concern. This book provides a simple, naturalistic method of locating and establishing the optimal pitch. New ways are utilized to develop the speaking voice with directed guidance given to the patient. Therapy is concentrated on the direct vocal rehabilitative process, i.e. changing the pitch, the tone focus, the quality, the volume, and breath support for speech. A modern automated method of practice using replay and naturalistic techniques for carry-over of these vocal elements have been developed and are described. Vocal psychotherapy, or the changing of the vocal image and the vocal identity that the patient has long maintained, associate therapy, illustrative therapy, and bibliotherapy, which have been devised as integral parts of therapy, are presented.

The techniques described in this book have produced excellent results for those undergoing vocal rehabilitation. Techniques, however, frequently are only as good as the person's skill in using them. Clinical vocal rehabilitation requires considerable insight and understanding of behavior. The voice therapist must be acutely aware of the effects that culture and society have upon the individual and his voice. Many voice patients have a *vocal* neurosis rooted in a society which has encouraged, developed, and sanctioned a vocal image, a vocal image which may result in a low-pitched voice and consequent vocal disorders. Thus, many who experience voice disorders require direct voice therapy to eliminate the dysphonia, vocal education to gain insight into the vocal myths surrounding the speaking voice, and vocal psychotherapy to alter the vocal image and vocal role.

CONTENTS

Part 5

VOCAL REHABILITATION:
OBSERVATIONS AND RESULTS

MODERN TECHNIQUES
OF
VOCAL REHABILITATION

PART 1

VOICE DISORDERS:
SYMPTOMS AND CAUSES

VOCAL REHABILITATION

Vocal rehabilitation is a recent discipline which concerns itself with the production or misproduction of the speaking voice and of the singing voice. The term "vocal rehabilitation" refers to the training or retraining of the following parameters of voice: pitch, tone focus, quality, volume, breath support, and rate.

Vocal rehabilitation is often inherent as an integral part in resolving functional and organic dysphonias. In functional dysphonia, no organic or neurological activating factor or factors is present. Vocal misuse and/or abuse is occurring within a normal laryngeal structure. Functional dysphonia includes the following categories: falsetto voice, ventricular phonation, nasality (functional), incipient spastic dysphonia and spastic dysphonia, hysterical dysphonia, hysterical aphonia and functional aphonia, bowed vocal folds (functional), and the largest category which this author terms "functional misphonia." Functional misphonia is a specific term which actually means functional "wrong voice." Functional misphonia defines a tired, hoarse, or weak voice without organic or neurological involvement, excluding the specific types listed above. General terms which encompass functional misphonia include chronic, nonspecific laryngitis (Baker), hyperkinetic and hypokinetic dysphonia (Arnold), phonasthenia (Flatau), hyperfunctional and hypofunctional dysphonia (Froeschels), executive dysphonia (Gardner), and aggravated voice (Tarneaud.)

Organic dysphonias include the following major categories and subcategories: (1) growths and lesions on the vocal folds, such as nodules, polyps, contact ulcer granuloma and/or fossa, polypoid degeneration, papillomatosis, keratosis, and leukoplakia; (2) structural anomalies, such as cleft or insufficient velar-pharyngeal closure creating nasality (organic) and bowed vocal folds (organic); (3) neurological, direct and indirect involvement, such as vocal fold paralysis (direct involvement), Parkinson's disease, postcoronary voice, multiple sclerosis, and amytrophic lateral sclerosis (indirect and direct involvement); (4) partial and

5

complete excision of the larynx, such as partial cordectomy, complete cordectomy, hemilaryngectomy, and laryngectomy. (Laryngectomy requires the specialized skill of esophageal speech training.) With the exception of laryngectomy, vocal misuse and abuse are usually occurring within the organically altered laryngeal structure in most organic dysphonias.

During the past ten years 1406 patients have been seen for voice evaluations and/or vocal rehabilitation by this author. This nonselective group includes 693 patients with functional dysphonia (486 functional misphonia, 34 falsetto, 11 ventricular phonation, 9 hysterical aphonia, 9 hysterical dysphonia, 5 functional aphonia, 42 spastic dysphonia, 21 incipient spastic dysphonia, 44 nasality [functional], and 32 bowed vocal folds [functional]). It also includes 713 patients with organic dysphonia (254 nodules, 68 polyps, 63 polypoid degeneration, 85 contact ulcers, 25 papillomata, 17 leukoplakia, 6 keratosis, 11 nasality [organic], 10 bowed vocal folds [organic], 59 paralytic dysphonias, 14 Parkinson's disease, 33 neurological [other], 3 partial cordectomies, 5 complete cordectomies, 5 hemilaryngectomies, and 55 laryngectomies). Extensive case histories have been charted and tabulated for these patients regarding vocal misuse and abuse, negative vocal symptoms of dysphonias, and the results of vocal rehabilitation. For an abbreviated overview of findings relevant to various aspects of vocal rehabilitation, two large groups of patients have been fully charted for discussion throughout the book. These two large groups are functional misphonia (486 patients) and organic dysphonia (470 patients), which includes nodules (254), polyps (68), polypoid degeneration (63), and contact ulcers (85). The two groupings total 956 patients.

SYMPTOMS OF FUNCTIONAL AND ORGANIC DYSPHONIAS

The negative vocal symptoms of functional and organic dysphonias may be categorized into three major groupings: sensory, auditory, and visual. Sensory symptoms are those sensations experienced by the patient which may activate him to seek medical assistance and/or vocal rehabilitation. Auditory symptoms are noted by either the patient (speaker) and/or the listener.

Visual symptoms are essentially confined to a laryngoscopic examination, direct or indirect. Dysphonic patients may experience one or more of these negative vocal symptoms in each of the three groupings.

Sensory Symptoms

The sensory symptoms include nonproductive throat clearing, coughing, progressive vocal fatigue following brief or extended vocal use; acute or chronic irritation or pain in or about larynx or pharynx; sternum pressure and/or pain; neck muscle cording; swelling of veins and/or arteries in the neck; throat stiffness; rapid vocal fatigue; feeling of a foreign substance or lump in the throat; ear irritation or tickling; repeated sore throats; a tickling, tearing, soreness, or burning sensation in the throat; scratchy or dry throat; tenderness of anterior and/or posterior strap muscles; rumble in chest; stinging sensation in soft palate; a feeling that talking is an effort; a choking feeling; tension and/or tightness in the throat; earache; back neck tension; headache; mucus formation; tracheal pressure; arytenoid tenderness; anterior or posterior cervical pain; pain at the base of the tongue; and chronic toothache without apparent cause.

The most common symptoms which patients complained about were vocal fatigue (functional misphonia, 448 patients or 92%; organic dysphonia, 441 patients or 94%); throat clearing (functional misphonia, 296 patients or 61%; organic dysphonia, 306 patients or 65%); and coughing (functional misphonia, 80 patients or 16%; organic dysphonia, 71 patients or 15%).

Vocal fatigue is the major sensory negative vocal symptom which indicates a functional or organic dysphonia. Unfortunately, vocal fatigue or tired voice is considered normal and seldom, if ever, does the individual experiencing this symptom realize that he is misusing his voice. If long-term vocal misuse and abuse are present, the patient may no longer be experiencing negative sensory symptoms, since he has become insensitive to the discomfort or pain.

Auditory Symptoms

Auditory symptoms include acute or chronic hoarseness; reduced or limited vocal range; inability to talk at will and at length in variable situations without experiencing impairment or loss of voice; tone change from a clear voice to a breathy, raspy, squeaky, foggy, or rough voice; repeated loss of voice; laryngitis; voice breaks; voice skips; voice which comes and goes during the day or over a period of months; clear voice in the morning with tired or foggy voice in the afternoon or evening; missed or inaudible speech sounds.

The most common auditory negative vocal symptom is hoarseness. Of the 956 patients seen, 440 or 91 percent of functional misphonic patients and 442 or 94 percent of organic dysphonic patients complained of hoarseness. Levin (1962) writes that hoarseness is the basic symptom which brings the patient to the physician.

Visual Symptoms

In functional dysphonias, a laryngoscopic examination may reveal redness, inflammation, or an edema of the vocal folds. In some cases, no apparent indications of vocal fold irritation or irregularity are present; however, these patients are usually experiencing sensory and/or auditory symptoms of the dysphonia. In organic dysphonias, the laryngologist will diagnose the disorder, such as thickening of the vocal folds, growths or lesions on the vocal folds, bowed vocal folds, paresis or paralyzed vocal fold, among other neurological involvements.

Functional dysphonias almost always exhibit auditory symptoms, usually present sensory symptoms, and may reveal visual symptoms. Organic dysphonias fundamentally present auditory, sensory, and visual symptoms.

VOCAL MISUSE AND ABUSE

Vocal misuse is defined as the use of an incorrect pitch, tone focus, quality, volume, breath support, and rate, either discretely or in combinations. By vocal abuse is meant the mistreatment of the vocal folds, as well as the laryngeal and pharyngeal musculature, by shouting, screaming, or talking in competition with noise, i.e. talking above, under, around, or through noise. As Clerf (1952, p. 6) states: "I know of no organ or structure in the whole body that is more abused than the larynx."

Vocal rehabilitation alleviates or eliminates vocal misuse and abuse by identifying and utilizing the correct pitch level and tone focus, developing proper breath support, using adequate volume, utilizing an acceptable quality and rate of voice, uncovering the etiological factors causing and continuing the voice disorder, utilizing vocal psychotherapy for comprehension of the vocal image, vocal role, and vocal identity, stressing and teaching good vocal hygiene, and mastering the production of the correct voice in all situations. A major concern of vocal rehabilitation is the vocal image, a concept that has been ignored or minimized. The vocal image is one of the most vital, pervasive, meaningful, and controlling factors in the onset, development, and resolution of voice disorders.

Vocal misuse and abuse are nearly always insidious in the onset and development with the initial stages of these conditions often unrecognized and untreated by vocal rehabilitation. They are frequently maltreated by palliative measures.

Vocal misuse is usually chronic, ranging from mild to severe in form, rather than ranging from acute to chronic which is the popular but incorrect belief. Vocal abuse may be acute or it may be chronic. For most individuals vocal abuse is an acute condition. It occurs during occasional situations such as ball games, parties, conferences, and airplane travel. The increased volume needed to talk above the noise level of these situations creates excessive laryngeal and pharyngeal tension. The pitch level used is too low or too high. Misuse of the pitch level heightens the vocal abuse. Shouting or screaming at ball games or parties also creates a similar condition of laryngeal and pharyngeal irritation. Shouting is abusive but not pathological unless it is a repeated procedure.

Some individuals experience chronic vocal abuse. Those who live and/or work in a noisy environment are consistently talking above, around, under, and through noise. These would include the mother with small children, the employee in a factory, the commuter on subways, buses, trains, cars, and planes, airport employees or those who live close to airports, the teacher supervising on a playground, construction workers, referees and umpires at ball games, and others in similar situations and occupations.

Chronic abuse can also be activated by anxieties and tensions so that an individual may shout or scream in an environment that is not essentially noisy. This type of abuse represents personality needs and demands of the individual as well as poor vocal knowledge and vocal usage. Examples of this type are the mother who is needlessly shouting at her child or children, the teacher who carries over the vociferous vocal pattern from the playground to the classroom, and the businessman who underscores his every thought with an exaggerated burst of volume.

Vocal abuse is often a habit so natural to a speaker or patient that he is unable to realize the activity of shouting is adverse and highly critical to his larynx and especially to his vocal folds. Loudness is a necessary catharsis for most persons at specific times but should not be used as a routine activity.

Vocal abuse may predispose or precipitate vocal misuse. An episode of acute vocal abuse may create inflammation of the vocal folds as well as irritation of laryngeal and pharyngeal muscles. This condition may produce hoarseness and cause the individual to use a decreased volume and a lower pitch level. The vocal folds may become edematous or thickened because of acute or chronic vocal abuse. The subsequent result is that the lowered pitch, which is inherent in this type of voice, may become a set vocal pattern, not only during hoarseness but also following the elimination of hoarseness.

Vocal misuse and abuse may be characterized by three stages, moving from mild to severe in symptomatology: sensory, auditory, and visual. Patients may experience one or more symptoms in each symptom grouping.

The first stage. *Sensory:* slight pain or irritation after prolonged vocal usage, some tension in or about the larynx or pharynx, mild mucus flow, some scratchy or itchy sensation within the larynx or pharynx, infrequent throat clearing, and an occasional sore throat. *Auditory:* slight hoarseness, mild laryngitis, some reduction in carrying power, thinning of voice as day progresses, some restriction in vocal range. *Visual:* inflammation or redness of vocal folds.

The second stage. *Sensory:* frequent throat clearing, increased tension in or about the larynx or pharynx, irritation in the larynx or pharynx, periodic sore throats, a feeling that speech is an effort, vocal fatigue after fairly brief vocal usage. *Auditory:* moderate hoarseness, some voice breaks or skips, periodic laryngitis, reduced vocal range, episodic loss of voice, more pronounced vocal impairment throughout the day. *Visual:* thickened or edematous vocal folds, incipient vocal nodules, polyps, or contact ulcer granuloma, slight bowing of vocal folds.

The third stage. *Sensory:* quick vocal fatigue after brief vocal usage, a feeling of a foreign substance or lump in the throat, consistent nonproductive throat clearing, effortful speech, irritation or pain in the larynx or pharynx, excessive mucus flow, recurrent sore throats, rumble in the chest, severe tension in the throat. *Auditory:* recurrent hoarseness and/or laryngitis, repeated voice breaks and skips, marked reduction in vocal range, repeated loss of voice, noticeable difficulty in being understood, evident lack of carrying power, voice failure occurring earlier in the day. *Visual:* growths or lesions on the vocal folds, pronounced bowing of the vocal folds, paralyzed vocal fold.

CAUSES OF VOCAL MISUSE AND ABUSE

Vocal misuse and abuse are usually due to a lack of correct vocal knowledge, a lack of proper vocal training, poor vocal models, emotional difficulties, and/or psychological problems. Brodnitz (1962, p. 455) writes: "Technically, the lack of proper instruction during professional training in the use of the speaking voice is responsible for many voice disorders." West, Ansberry, and Carr (1957, p. 76) state: "(No amount of vigorous vocalization can damage the edges of the vocal folds if the voice is properly used.)"

Nearly all voice patients seen have inept vocal concepts regarding the proper use of the speaking and/or singing voice. Vocal rehabilitation should alter misguided vocal concepts into meaningful vocal patterns, should include specialized vocal training to meet individual vocal needs, should provide practice in proper vocal usage, and should afford a new vocal image and vocal identity, thereby eliminating the causes of vocal misuse and abuse.

RESULTS OF VOCAL MISUSE AND ABUSE

Vocal misuse and abuse are fundamental factors in the creation and development of almost all functional dysphonias and most organic dysphonias, with the exception of neurological involvement, structural irregularities (congenital or acquired), and partial or complete excision of the larynx. Vocal misuse and abuse, however, may develop as a consequence of neurological involvement and partial laryngeal excision or may be superimposed on these organic conditions. McClosky (1959, p. 73) indicates: "The vast majority of patients who have come to me for voice therapy have been suffering from vocal abuse, that is to say, misuse."

The major type of functional dysphonia which is created and maintained by vocal misuse and abuse is functional misphonia. With continued vocal misuse and abuse, functional misphonia may develop into benign organic lesions of the vocal folds.

Vocal misuse and abuse are fundamental productive factors in the creation of nodes, polyps, and polypoid degeneration according to Friedberg and Segall (1941) (polyps and polypoid degeneration), Ash and Schwartz (1944) (nodes and polyps), Holinger and Johnston (1951) (nodes and polyps), Kelly and Craik (1952) (nodes), Brodnitz (1958) (nodules), Wilson (1962a and 1962b) (nodules), Baker (1962) (nodules), O'Neil and McGee (1962) (polyps), Arnold (1962d and 1963b) (nodules and polyps), Baker (1963) (polypoid degeneration), and Fisher and Logemann (1970) (nodules).

Contact ulcer fossa and contact ulcer granuloma are directly related to vocal misuse and abuse by Jackson (1928), Jackson and Jackson (1935a), Peacher (1947a, 1947b, 1947c, and 1961), Peacher and Holinger (1947), New and Devine (1949), Baker (1954), Holinger and Johnston (1960), von Leden and Moore (1960), Levin (1962), Brodnitz (1963), Myerson (1964), and Cooper and Nahum (1967).

Vocal misuse and abuse must be considered as possible etiological factors in the onset of acute and/or chronic laryngitis, of premalignant lesions of the vocal folds, such as papillomata, leukoplakia, and keratosis or hyperkeratosis, and of carcinoma of the vocal folds. Clerf (1937) and Murphy (1967) write that acute and/or chronic laryngitis may be caused by vocal misuse and/or abuse. Greene (1964, p. 91) states: "Chronic laryngitis and sore throats are frequently the result of bad habits of voice production."* Gabriel and Jones (1960) report that vocal abuse (among other irritants) caused chronic laryngitis, and in 51 cases of cancer of the larynx, 19.7 percent initially had chronic laryngitis.

The theoretical foundation of the development of premalignant growths, such as keratosis, leukoplakia, and papillomata, to malignant growths is posited by this author as follows: (1) The misuse and abuse of the speaking voice creates inflammation and irritation of the vocal folds without organic damage. This irritation and inflammation may be acute, but with repeated damage to the folds by continued vocal misuse and abuse, along with other irritants such as smoking, the inflammation and irritation become chronic and move into the next stage. (2) Thickening or edema of the folds takes place. This stage may also be acute or chronic. The thickening, or hyperplasia, in time with continued vocal misuse and abuse, turns to metaplasia. (3) Benign growths such as nodules, polyps, and contact ulcers may follow continued vocal misuse; the growths may then progress into the premalignant growths, such as leukoplakia, keratosis, and papillomata. Or the premalignant growths may develop directly from the metaplasia, circumventing the benign growth stage. These premalignant growths remain within the acute or chronic stage before moving on to malignancy. It is posited that this stage is reversible or can be stagnated by vocal rehabilitation plus the cessation of other irritants, such as smoking. (4) Malignant growths occur on the vocal folds.

All the stages herein described do not occur in each individual; some stages progress more rapidly than others (again with individual variation), and some stages remain more static than others. Knowledge of such stage development would be helpful, if not vital, in determining when vocal misuse and abuse must

---

* M. Greene, *The Voice and Its Disorders*, 2nd ed. London, Pitman Medical Publishing Co., 1964.

cease, if such a factor is contributory and pertinent to the onset and development of vocal fold cancer.

The theory that vocal misuse and abuse create or contribute to the onset and development of vocal fold malignancy remains a theory presently supported in the most part by clinical experience and some research.

Jackson and Jackson (1939, p. 210) write: "The location of 85 percent of cancers on the most abused part of the larynx, the middle third of the cord, renders it logical, even if not probable, that vocal abuse is one cause of cancer of the larynx."* Cavanaugh (1923) says that laryngeal irritation predisposes to malignancy. Tucker (1935 and 1937) finds that chronic irritation may be one factor in the change from benign growths to malignant growths. Mitchell (1943, p. 250) says: "Benign tumors cannot be overlooked as a factor in the production of cancer." Froeschels (1943, p. 129) writes: "The pressure of one vocal cord against the other in production of the *coup de glotte* may even favor a malignant growth in a predisposed person." Wallner (1954, p. 260) reports: "Speaking with chronically inflamed vocal cords may lead to voice strain that results in the formation of polyps or of polypoid degeneration. The prolonged irritation of the mucosa may cause keratosis or even malignancy."

Pietrantoni and Fior (1958), in studying 200 unselected patients with cancer of the larynx, have found that 14 percent of their cases suffered from voice strain. They feel that these findings indicated that voice strain was important in the genesis of cancer of the larynx. Luse (1965) has reviewed the occupations of 491 laryngectomees prior to surgery. Their occupations had involved trauma of the vocal folds from pulling, pushing, lifting, or from vocal abuse. Many of the patients had had to talk in noise on their jobs.

Vocal misuse and abuse are linked with papilloma, leukoplakia, and hyperkeratosis. Brewer and Briess (1960a, p. 462) write:

Screamers, speakers, or singers nodes have long been reckoned as

---

* C. Jackson and C. L. Jackson, *Cancer of the Larynx*. Philadelphia, W. B. Saunders, 1939.

the wages of voice strain, yet many swollen vocal cords without other evidences of inflammation, polyps, papillomas in the adult, contact ulcers, hyperkeratoses, and leukoplakia, as well as localized
edemas and inflammatory areas, can now be traced to specific intrinsic laryngeal muscle dysfunction for their etiology.

Kernan (1937) notes the relationship between voice strain and
hematoma which lead to papilloma. Cracovaner (1965) writes
that if causal factors such as cigarette smoking, alcohol, and vocal abuse are eliminated, hyperkeratotic and leukoplakia lesions
may be reversed. Cooper (1971a) reports the results of a three-
month program of vocal rehabilitation for eight patients with
biopsied papillomas of the vocal folds. In four of the eight
subjects, laryngologists found that slight to extreme reductions
had occurred in the size of the lesions.

In summary, the results of vocal misuse and abuse are variable. They depend upon the circumstances, the degree and extent of the misuse, and the external and internal needs of or demands upon the individual.

Controlled research is limited in isolating the variables that
may produce cancer of the vocal folds through the stages previously described, with vocal misuse and abuse contributing to
all stages. The premalignant conditions of the vocal folds—
leukoplakia, keratosis, and papillomata—must be studied as to
the effect and results of vocal rehabilitation, as it eliminates the
vocal misuse and abuse.

OVERUSE OR EXCESSIVE USE OF THE
SPEAKING VOICE

Vocal misuse and abuse are often either confused with overuse of the voice or thought to be synonymous with vocal overuse, as mentioned by Ash and Schwartz (1944) (vocal misuse or
excess use) and Withers and Dawson (1960) (vocal misuse or
overuse). Vocal misuse and overuse or excessive use are two separate entities. Although overuse or excessive use of the voice is
usually listed as a leading cause of voice disorders, in reality,
misuse and abuse should be cited as basic causes.

Overuse of the speaking voice does not occur at any time unless the speaking voice is misused and abused. If vocal misuse

and abuse are transpiring, any use is overuse. There is no such condition as overuse of the speaking voice if the speaking voice is properly used. Overuse is a factor only when vocal rest is essential for healing following a surgical procedure, when the individual has a cold or upper respiratory infection which has adversely affected the vocal folds, or when the vocal parameters (pitch, tone focus, breath support) are influenced by a severe mental or physical condition. The term overuse is a misnomer. Voice disorders are not due to *overuse* of the voice; they are due to *misuse and abuse* of the voice. A voice well used is essentially never overused.

PITCH AND VOCAL MISUSE

Vocal misuse occurs most frequently in pitch. An optimal pitch level is one to three tones within an optimal pitch range (a series of notes surrounding the optimal pitch level) which affords the maximum amount of sound with the least amount of effort. The habitual pitch level is one to three tones within the habitual pitch range (a series of notes surrounding the habitual pitch level) which an individual uses during spontaneous speech. If the optimal and habitual pitch levels and ranges are identical, vocal misuse does not occur. If the habitual pitch differs from the optimal pitch, vocal misuse prevails. Most individuals do not utilize the optimal pitch range as their habitual pitch range.

A few authors indicate that a pitch which is too high contributes to dysphonias. West, Ansberry, and Carr (1957) and Van Riper and Irwin (1958) find that nodules are generally caused by too high a pitch, among other factors. Anderson (1961, p. 81) states: "Habitual use of a pitch level that is too high may produce vocal nodules." Voorhees (1914) writes that too high a pitch causes vocal fatigue in speakers. Jackson (1940) believes that myasthenia laryngis in speakers may be created by using too high a pitch.

The most frequent form of vocal misuse involving pitch is the use of too low a habitual pitch. This finding has been reported in the literature and is borne out by this author's clinical experience. Williamson (1945) finds that 69 out of 72 patients were speaking below their optimal pitch level. Gardner (1958,

p. 180) reports: "Practically all of the executives spoke below their respective normal levels of pitch." Hanley and Thurman (1962, p. 144) explain: "But far too many persons, in our experience, self-diagnose 'too high' (rarely 'too low' for either sex) pitch levels, set about lowering pitch, and by so doing perhaps lay the groundwork for future serious vocal disturbances."* Peacher (1966, p. 19) also finds: "Most people who have vocal problems will have to raise their pitch from two to five notes. This is contrary to the popular conception that a beautiful speaking voice is always low-pitched." Heinberg (1964, p. 185) writes: "So long as habitual pitch can be raised without resulting in a thin voice quality, the higher it is set, the better."†

Cornut and Cornut (1965) state that a low fundamental pitch was a symptom in 40 cases of dysphonia in women. Tarneaud (1947) defines that aggravated voice, a functional problem, has a lowered pitch, diminished intensity, and a husky quality. Boland (1953, p. 110) writes: "The obviously hoarse patient is usually speaking at the bottom of his pitch range, his pitch is a monotone, and he uses too much energy in speaking." Clinical experience indicates that the overwhelming majority of patients with functional dysphonias (except falsetto and hysterical aphonia) and most organic dysphonias, such as nodules, polyps, contact ulcers, leukoplakia, keratosis, and papillomata, are generally speaking at too low a pitch level.

A spectrographic analysis to determine fundamental frequencies before and after therapy for 155 dysphonic patients showed an increase in fundamental frequencies following therapy for 150 patients of the 155 patients (Cooper, 1972). These results indicated that 150 patients of this group were utilizing too low a pitch level prior to therapy, since the higher or optimal pitch level alleviated and/or eliminated the dysphonia and the negative vocal symptoms. The mean fundamental frequencies increased during therapy for all dysphonias except hysterical dysphonia and falsetto.

---

* Theodore Hanley and Wayne Thurman, *Developing Vocal Skills*. New York, Holt, Rinehart and Winston, 1962.

† Paul Heinberg, *Voice Training*, Copyright, 1964, Ronald Press Co., New York.

The speaking voice range in normal individuals is considered to be approximately one octave. Most individuals utilize a small segment of this range. Voice patients exhibit a limited range, usually the lower portion of the pitch range. Flower (1959) mentions that patients utilized usually only three or four tones at the lower end of the pitch range. Routine use of any pitch level without variation produces a monotone voice. Most monotone voices are the result of habitually using this limited lower pitch level. Heinberg (1964, p. 185) believes: *"The higher the habitual pitch level, the more pitch variety one uses, and vice versa."**

Some writers have indicated that singing at too high a pitch level may contribute to voice disorders, such as myasthenia laryngis (Jackson, 1940) and nodules (Brodnitz, 1958). Cunning (1934) notes that singing and speaking too low causes nodes. Children and adults who sing in choruses, choirs, or groups may be singing at pitch levels which are too high or too low. Clinical experience indicates that singing at a pitch level that is either too high or too low creates vocal pathology. Most of the patients seen who are singers with voice disorders have been speaking at too low a pitch level (Cooper, 1970c and 1970k).

Basal Pitch

Many individuals are utilizing a basal or near basal pitch level as the habitual pitch. The basal pitch is defined by Van Riper and Irwin (1958, p. 300) as: "the lowest note on which [one] . . . can sustain utterance."† The use of the basal or near basal pitch, which could be referred to as the basal pitch range, creates dysphonias. Of 486 functional misphonic patients seen and 470 organic dysphonic patients seen, 441 or 91 percent of functional misphonia and 432 or 92 percent of organic dysphonia were using habitual pitch ranges which approximated the basal pitch ranges.

Cooper and Yanagihara (1971) found that the basal pitch

* Paul Heinberg, *Voice Training*, Copyright, 1964, Ronald Press Co., New York.

† Charles Van Riper and John V. Irwin, *Voice and Articulation*, p. 300. Copyright 1958, Prentice-Hall, Englewood Cliffs, New Jersey.

level fluctuates throughout the day. The basal pitch was lowest in the morning in almost all subjects studied. This pitch level rose one to three semitones during the day, rising more in some than in others. For some subjects, the rise continued until afternoon; in others, the pitch dropped from noon to afternoon.

Occasionally, the vocal fry is used as part of the normal speech pattern. According to Michel (1968), the vocal fry is extremely low in pitch with a mean fundamental frequency of 36.4 hertz. Hollien, Moore, Wendahl, and Michel (1966, p. 246) define the vocal fry as a "phonational register occurring at frequencies below those of the modal register." Clinical observations have indicated that the vocal fry is far below the basal pitch level. Although the vocal fry may be classified experimentally as the lowest portion of the range, when this author refers to the lowest portion of the pitch range, he is referring to the basal pitch range.

Hollien, Moore, Wendahl, and Michel (1966, p. 246) note:

> It should not be inferred from the previous discussion, however, that vocal fry cannot be present in, or as, a vocal pathology. It is probably true that, if an individual phonates only in the vocal fry mode, he has a voice disorder—just as an individual who can speak only in falsetto has a voice disorder. It is simply our intent to suggest that ordinarily vocal fry constitutes one of several physiologically available types of voice production on the frequency-pitch continuum and hence, of itself, is not logically classified among the laryngeal pathologies. Stated somewhat differently, while the excessive use of fry could result in a diagnosis of voice disorder, this quality is too often heard in normal voices (especially in descending inflections where the voice fundamental falls below frequencies sustainable in the modal register) to be exclusively a disorder. In sum it is difficult to conceive that this very common vocal quality does, in fact, result solely from laryngeal pathologies.

Hollien and Wendahl (1968) indicate that because of the low frequency and the perceptual regularity of the vocal fry, it is not classified among vocal pathologies. Clinically, the vocal fry is a pathology, since continued use of the vocal fry creates the same pathological condition as continued use of the basal pitch level and range. This author would agree that the vocal fry, used sparingly and intermittently, is a routine part of some speaking patterns. The continued use of such a pattern does not make it utilitarian nor nonpathological just as continued use of the basal or near basal pitch does not make it utilitarian nor nonpathological.

The basal pitch level and/or range is utilized in two main types of voices: the low-pitched vocal image voice (Cooper, 1969a) and the "morning voice" (Perkins, 1957, p. 865) or "post-sleep voice" (Ladefoged, 1964). The basal pitch level or range may also be utilized during illness, mental depression, physical disability, and physical or mental fatigue, as discussed under contributory factors of vocal misuse.

The low-pitched voice utilized by most voice patients is largely the result of the vocal image. The vocal image, which is fully discussed later, may be developed through vocal stereotypes which are perpetuated by the vocal culture and the mass media of communication (Cooper, 1969a, 1970n).

The morning or post-sleep voice utilizes a basal or near basal pitch level due to the relaxed state of the individual's muscular system, especially the laryngeal musculature, following a period of sleep. The morning voice has been investigated as a clinical entity through patient questionnaires and through research. The questionnaires have revealed that 71 percent of both the 486 functional misphonic and the 470 organic dysphonic patients have experienced a basal or near basal pitch level or range upon arising in the morning. Cooper (1965), in an unpublished study, has investigated the habitual pitch of normal speakers (seven females and six males) by testing the habitual pitch three times daily for two days. After determining the average habitual pitch for the morning, for noon, and for the afternoon, he has found that the average habitual pitch was lowest in the morning in both female and male subjects.

The low-pitched morning voice may be clear or it may be hoarse. Russell (1936, p. 114) describes a hoarseness or heavy quality to the voice upon awakening, which is normal. Clinical findings indicate that the hoarseness may disappear as the voice is used or as the individual becomes physically active.

The key factor in the morning voice is that it is pitched at the basal or near basal pitch level or range. When the pitch of the morning voice is continued, it is productive of vocal pathology.

Perkins (1957), on the other hand, recommends use of the morning voice since it is the most relaxed voice. Cooper (1971c) finds that since the morning voice utilizes only the bottom portion of the total pitch range, it should not be used routinely or continuously. The tone focus of the low-pitched morning voice is almost always located within the laryngopharynx, instead of within the oronasolaryngopharynx. Continued use of the pitch level and tone focus inherent in the morning voice creates pharyngeal and laryngeal tensions, lacks carrying power, flexibility, durability, and easy intelligibility, and requires increased volume for production.

TONE FOCUS AND VOCAL MISUSE

Tone focus is the emphasis or placement of resonance in one or more portions of the throat or pharynx. The three major areas of resonance are the laryngopharynx (lower throat resonance), the oropharynx (middle throat or mouth area), and the nasopharynx (upper throat or nose area). All voices have laryngopharyngeal resonance, since the sound must be emitted through this resonating chamber.

Most patients with voice disorders incur vocal misuse by emphasizing or stressing laryngopharyngeal resonance which results in pharyngeal and laryngeal tensions. These tensions cause the patient to experience negative sensory and auditory vocal symptoms. Too much tone focus in the laryngopharynx results in a gutteral voice; too much tone focus in the oropharynx results in a flat, colorless, or denasal voice; too much tone focus in the nasopharynx results in a nasal voice.

Correct tone focus is the balance of oral and nasal resonance with some laryngeal resonance. This tone placement is achieved by focusing or directing the tone to the "mask" (an area which includes the bridge and sides of the nose down to and around the lips). Laryngopharyngeal resonance is natural and need not be emphasized.

QUALITY AND VOCAL MISUSE

The quality of voice may be affected by the following factors, among others: an incorrect tone focus, a poor pitch level or range, and/or an impairment of the vocal folds, all of which may be functional or organic in nature. Conditions, such as allergies, sinusitis, and postnasal drip, may create changes in the vocal folds and mucous membrane of the pharynx, which in turn may affect the quality of voice. The main vocal quality deviations include nasality, hoarseness, harshness, and breathiness. Additional terms are often used to describe these qualities or combinations of these qualities.

Quality is closely related to pitch and tone focus. Holmes (1930) writes that a suitable pitch level and correct tonal placement are needed for good vocal quality. Flower (1959) states that a clear fluid vocal tone usually results in an approximate optimal pitch.

A nasal quality or a strident quality is produced by an unbalanced tone focus, one that has too much nasopharyngeal placement. Hypernasal speech may be produced by many factors. One of these is functional nasality in which there is no organic or neurological abnormality; the palatal and pharyngeal muscles are simply not being used to close the velar pharyngeal port. Functional nasality may be caused by imitiation of poor vocal models, among other factors.

Hypernasal speech may also be produced by organic or neurological factors, such as a cleft palate, or a submucous cleft palate, neurological impairments of muscles controlling the nasopharyngeal port, or anatomical abnormalities. In some cases a tonsillectomy and adenoidectomy may create an organic or neurological nasality. Hoopes, Dellon, Fabrikant, and Soliman (1970, p. 50), in studying hypernasality, summarize: "The diagnosis of neurogenic hypernasal speech cannot be applied indiscriminately to all patients not demonstrating an overt or submucous cleft palate. Cineradiographic analysis can identify subtle but discrete anatomical abnormalities capable of producing hypernasal speech."

Vocal fold growths, such as nodules, polyps, or contact ulcer granulomas, as well as inflamed vocal folds, may be secondary and minor factors in the creation of an impaired vocal quality, depending upon the size, extent, and portion of the growth(s) on the vocal folds. Hoarseness, breathiness, and harshness may be created by laryngopharyngeal tone focus and by a basal or near basal pitch level. Williamson (1945, p. 201), in a review of the relationship between pitch and hoarseness, finds: "The most common principal cause of hoarse-voice was the throat tension resulting from the effort to speak at a level far below optimal pitch."

Hoarseness is the most prevalent clinical voice quality. Boland (1953, p. 109) states:

> . . . *the number of persons who are being treated for hoarseness is infinitesimal compared to the number of people who need treatment.*
>
> . . .
>
> An individual's opinion about his own voice may not be reliable. People who are hoarse often think of their own voices as being "mellow" or "deep and resonant."

Lieberman (1963) writes that listeners could not easily identify hoarseness unless they knew the speaker's normal voice. Lieberman also says that a speaker's estimate of his hoarseness is probably related to the extent of soreness he is feeling.

When the optimal pitch level is located and the tone focus is balanced in the oronasopharynx, the quality usually becomes normal or near normal. Only when the inflammation is extremely severe or the growth(s) are very large and impede the closure of the vocal folds is it difficult to achieve a normal or near normal vocal quality. Unilateral or bilateral growths seldom impair vocal quality if the proper pitch level and tone focus are utilized. Polypoid degeneration of the vocal folds does not easily afford the maintenance of the correct pitch level and tone focus; therefore, the quality often remains impaired when this growth is present.

A spectrographic analysis to determine the degree of hoarseness present in 3 vowels of 27 dysphonic patients before and after therapy showed all patients displaying hoarseness in varying degrees in the vowels prior to therapy. Following therapy, these patients were basically free of hoarseness; only a trace of or slight hoarseness was seen within one vowel in a few patients (Cooper, 1972).

VOLUME AND VOCAL MISUSE

Vocal misuse may occur if the volume is excessive or if the volume is inadequate. In these dysphonic patients, because of the use of the basal or near basal pitch level and of the tone focus within the laryngopharynx, both excessive volume and inadequate volume created laryngeal and pharyngeal tensions. These tensions, in combination with the misuse of pitch and tone focus, the vocal image, and personality factors, resulted in functional or organic dysphonias. Usually, excessive volume heightens the dysphonia more rapidly and more actively than inadequate volume. Inadequate volume, when the sound is forced, can also instigate functional and organic dysphonias. Inadequate volume has the additional problem of lack of intelligibility.

Volume tends to increase when a distracting noise level increases (Hanley and Steer, 1949). Voice problems may be created by competition with industrial noise (Brewer & Briess, 1960b). The noise level at cocktail parties may reach a maximum level of 80-85dB (Legget and Northwood, 1960).

Individuals who abuse the voice frequently by yelling, by shouting, or by talking above noise may create or contribute to functional and organic dysphonias. Those individuals who only infrequently participate in any vocal abuse of the type described above may not experience a voice problem per se unless they are already misusing their voices (incorrect pitch and tone focus). If the voice is being misused, any type of intensive or excessive misuse or abuse may result in a more severe functional misphonia or in an organic dysphonia.

BREATH SUPPORT AND VOCAL MISUSE

Many dysphonic patients utilize an incorrect type of breathing for speech, such as upper chest or clavicular breathing. In upper chest breathing, the upper portion of the chest moves in and out. In clavicular breathing, the shoulders move up and down. These two forms of breathing create laryngeal, pharyngeal, and bodily tensions.

The most efficient and effective type of breathing which should be routinely used for both speech and for vegetative purposes is midsection breath support. Midsection breath support is also known as medial, abdominal, diaphragmatic, or central breathing. In this type of breathing the midsection or abdomen moves smoothly and imperceptibly in and out. Midsection breath support involves the concept of midsection breath control. Some individuals use different types of breathing for vegetative purposes as opposed to speech. Others may use combinations of these types of breathing for vegetative purposes and for speech.

Clinically, it has been found that the lack of midsection breath support has initiated or abetted the onset and development of the dysphonia. Of the patients seen, 418 or 86 percent of functional misphonic and 420 or 89 percent of organic dysphonic patients had upper chest or clavicular breathing.

Brodnitz (1962, p. 466) writes: "The prevalence of chest breathing is very frequent in disturbed voices." He also states (p. 475): "The treatment of almost any voice disorder requires correction of the breathing habits of the patient." Moore (1957, p. 694) points out: "There can be little doubt that many persons with harmful vocal habits expend more effort on breathing than is necessary."

Studies edited by Gray (1936) find specific types of breathing are unrelated to audibility (Sallee, 1936) and to loudness (Wiksell, 1936). These studies were laboratory experiments which were not concerned with ongoing speech. Continuous speech of necessity requires proper breath support from the midsection. This has been conclusively demonstrated clinically in the vast majority of patients seen. Not only is midsection breath support necessary for continuous audibility and loudness in spontaneous conversational speech, but it is also vital to avoid laryngeal and pharyngeal tensions as well as bodily tensions produced by other types of breath support. Midsection breath support is also necessary to provide flexible breath control. In a fluoroscopic study of good and poor speakers, Huyck and Allen (1937) note that regular diaphragmatic movement is present in good voices. Midsection breath support allows for proper tone focus and optimal pitch, as well as providing for durability, comfort, and ease of voice.

RATE AND VOCAL MISUSE

Rate is a minor problem in the constellation of factors contributing to a functional dysphonia or an organic dysphonia.

Rate is considered in only two instances: (1) if the rate is so rapid that either labored breathing or hyperventilation occurs; or (2) if the rate is too fast to allow a patient to concentrate on the components of vocal rehabilitation, i.e. pitch, tone focus, and breath support. Rate that is too slow has seldom been encountered.

Rapid rate may be utilized to mask an accent, an articulation problem, and stuttering; a slow rate may also be used to contain stuttering. In some patients seen, rapid or slow rate has been expressive of a personality need, has been due to a habit developed from imitation or has been caused by a neurological impairment, such as cerebral palsy or oral apraxia.

PHYSICAL CONTRIBUTORY FACTORS TO VOCAL MISUSE AND ABUSE

A wide range of environmental and/or constitutional factors may contribute to vocal misuse and abuse. Some of these are smoking, air conditioning, smog, chlorine water, food, allergies, postnasal drip, sinusitis, infected tonsils, deviated septum, hormones, premenstrual tensions, pregnancy, menopause, upper respiratory infections or colds, coughing, and bodily fatigue.

Smoking has a marked tendency to lower the pitch due possibly to a thickening of the vocal folds, and/or a relaxation of individual. The lowered pitch often creates vocal misuse. Smoking can be considered to be a direct cause of the onset and development of functional misphonia as well as organic dysphonias, involving both benign and premalignant lesions.

Climatic conditions influence some voices. Clinical experience reveals the speaking voice may be affected by smog. A limited number of voice patients report, too, that the lack of vocal control due to a long period in air conditioning, as well as in and out of air conditioning, has contributed to their voice problem.

Food may have the tendency in some patients to impair the quality of voice as well as lower the pitch. A full meal relaxes the body and may create a drowsiness.

Chlorine water affects the voice (Manser, 1939). Some patients report difficulty in controlling the pitch as well as presenting a veiled or impaired quality of voice during or after swimming.

The intubation process may infrequently create vocal fold irritation or inflammation or a growth on the vocal folds, such as a nodule, a polyp, or a contact ulcer granuloma, or may cause paralysis of the vocal folds. Intubation is a medical procedure in which a tube is inserted between the vocal folds during anesthesia. The intubation may be necessary for a surgical procedure or for a direct laryngoscopy.

Many writers have discussed the various problems caused by intubation. Some of these authors include El-Mofti (1949) (polypoid growths), Corbetta and Felletti (1961) (granuloma), Kürthy (1966) (granuloma), Bergström (1964) (granuloma), Farrior (1942) (contact ulcer), Harrison and Tonkin (1967) (laryngeal complications), and Yamashita (1965) (paralysis). Lu, Tamura, and Koobs (1961), who outline cases of laryngeal pathology following endotracheal anesthesia, also present a bibliography of 34 articles. Bergström, Moberg, and Orell (1962) call attention to the fact that after about twenty hours of intubation, extensive ulcerations occur in the larynx. Baron and Kohlmoos (1951, p. 789) report "that important laryngeal sequelae can occur from endotracheal anesthesia in both adults and children and that they are not uncommon in children." However, Harrison and Tonkin (1967, p. 606) state: "In the majority of cases in which granulomas of the vocal cords or oedema of the arytenoids is present, spontaneous improvement occurs." Zilstorff (1968, p. 1150) comments: "Alterations in the voice have been observed following intubation anaesthesia, often a loss of high tones or difficulty in equalizing the tones." Farrior (1942, p. 239) reaches the following conclusions:

1. The delicate mucous membrane overlying the vocal process of the arytenoid cartilage is susceptible to injury by the intratracheal cannula.

2. Hoarseness developing after intratracheal anesthesia warrants repeated laryngeal examinations.

König (1967) discusses upper laryngeal lesions created by feeding tubes. These tubes may injure the mucosal lining and, because of the continuous pressure exerted on the laryngeal cartilages, may result in edema and perichondritis. Ankylosis of the cricoarytenoid joint occurred in one case.

Postintubation voice problems are not common. These problems fall into two categories. The first group includes vocal fold irritation or a growth which disappears following vocal rest. The other group involves the continuation of the inflammation or the growth due to vocal misuse and abuse. This vocal misuse may have been present prior to the intubation, or the trauma to the vocal folds may have created an inability to control the vocal folds during vocalization and thus the patient began a pattern of vocal misuse. This latter group can benefit from vocal rehabilitation. Lack of attention to the dysphonia results in further vocal misuse and abuse and contributes to an ongoing cycle of vocal tension, misuse, and dysphonia.

Allergies, sinusitis, postnasal drip, and infected tonsils may all affect the voice by causing thickened vocal folds, swollen mucous membrane of the pharynx, and other conditions. The quality of voice may become breathy, hoarse, nasal or denasal. The pitch of the voice is usually lowered. The tone focus may become unbalanced either with too much nasal resonance or with too little nasal resonance combined with too much oral and laryngeal resonance. Some patients seen have reported relief from voice problems by a combination of vocal rehabilitation and medical treatment. Clinical experience has revealed that these conditions, although they may affect the voice, are without essential effect or control if the voice is used correctly and if the conditions are not excessive. If the individual is suffering from vocal misuse, these conditions will contribute to continued and heightened vocal misuse. Many patients suffering from these conditions have normal voices. A deviated septum, which is affecting the nasal intake of air and is in combination possibly with allergy, sinusitis, and/or excessive postnasal drip, may require surgical correction in order to provide a better air passage.

Hormonal effect upon the voice has been found to be minimal in patients seen who were taking thyroxin and estrogen. Testosterone and its derivatives have produced the most noticeable voice change in women, such as lowered pitch and hoarseness, which would be expected from the thickened vocal folds.

Some patients seen who were taking testosterone have responded to vocal rehabilitation once the hormonal extract was terminated.

Bauer (1963, 1968) notes the relationship of voice problems
to hormones and drugs. Imre (1965) frequently finds voice disorders among older patients taking hormones for climacteric
complaints or for carcinoma of the mammary glands or the
prostrate gland. Damste (1967) reports that 10 percent of 400
women with voice complaints had used a virilizing agent. He
(1964, 1967) treats the problem with vocal therapy; however, he
advises preventive treatment by avoidance of the hormones if
possible. The effect of anabolic steroids or testosterone on wom-
en's voices has also been noted by Goldman and Salmon (1942),
Bauer (1963), Calvet and Coll (1964), Grimaud and Bonneville
(1964), Damste (1964), and Van Deinse, Dieleman, and Drost
(1966). Brodnitz (1962, p. 281) observes: "Vocal quality is deeply influenced by changes in the metabolic and hormonal bal-
ances, and by the shifts between the two opposing forces of the
autonomic nervous system." In a recent publication, Brodnitz
(1971, p. 190) summarizes:

> Transitory voice changes during menstruation and in pregnancy
> are common. Irreversible voice changes may be produced by the
> administration of mixed hormones in the treatment of menopausal
> complaints. The widespread use of anabolic steroids has increased
> sharply the risk of permanent virilization of voice.

Some female patients have indicated that they experience
some difficulty with the voice, especially a lowered pitch, prior
to the menstrual period. Frable (1962) found premenstrual tension affected the voice through hoarseness, lowered vocal pitch,
and vocal instability. Wendler, Igel, and Steindel (1968, p. 247)
observed: "Vocal performance is often more less [sic] restricted
during menstruation. . . . Especially in persons with heavy vocal
disturbances before or during the normal menstruation we observed a distinctly lower reduction in performance during the
medicamentous interval."

van Thal (1961) reports that pitch and quality may be affected by pregnancy. Voorhees (1914) finds pregnancy and menstruation may affect quality and carrying power. A few patients seen

have reported that their voice problems dated from the time of pregnancy. However, a review of these patients reveals that they had vocal misuse, such as a lowered pitch, and a vocal image prior to the pregnancy. The pregnancy possibly exacerbated the condition.

Menopause has not found to be a serious or lasting impact upon the well-used voice. Patients who experienced any vocal difficulty at all which could possibly be linked to the menopause responded very well to vocal rehabilitation.

The patient must understand that the effect of hormones on the voice is twofold. One is the direct effect on the body, including the larynx, that the hormonal change has; the other is the indirect effect on the voice from the emotions which may have been affected by the hormones.

Another major influence on the voice is the upper respiratory infection or cold. This condition can also influence the voice through the emotions. Goldman (1967, p. 34) writes: "Some pneumonias of uncertain etiology ('non-specific,' or 'virus' pneumonias) and prolonged course, are often associated with severe emotional change, particularly depression, to the degree that a kind of vicious cycle is set up." Of course, the primary effect of the cold or upper respiratory infection is the direct one on the larynx and pharynx of thickened and irritated vocal folds, swollen mucous membrane, nasal discharge and many other variables. Meano (1967, p. 154) observes: "Any illness of the lungs and bronchi (bronchitis, pulmonitis, etc.) all too obviously interfere [*sic*] with sound production."

Cold or infection may be closely related to the misused voice, according to Froeschels (1943, p. 129) who writes:

> Hygiene of the voice may even prevent organic disorders of the respiratory tract. The epithelium of the vocal cords, as well as that of the mucous linings of the throat, is injured by the continuous attack due to a hyperfunctional state and therefore may be more susceptible to infection.

Moses (1954, p. 6) writes:

> The energy potential of an individual may be lowered during or after some acute disease and this could make vocal expression taxing. . . . Acute localized diseases can render functioning of the larynx

difficult for a time and the individual can develop inefficient use of his larynx during this period and retain these habits after the acute condition disappears.*

A cold or an upper respiratory infection may serve as a precipitating factor in creating a voice disorder. Many voice patients have experienced these types of infections without encountering a voice problem; however, if any of the following factors occur, a voice disorder may result: (1) if the infection is particularly severe and/or prolonged; (2) if the infection occurs in combination with bodily fatigue and/or psychological depression; (3) if the individual attempts to protect or pamper his voice by speaking softer and unknowingly lowering the pitch; (4) if the individual likes the lowered pitch created by the cold. Because the individual uses the lowered pitch of voice during the protracted period of the infection, he may develop a new vocal pattern and a new vocal image, which continues after the cold has subsided. Unfortunately, this new voice with the lowered pitch is a misused voice which often results in a voice disorder.

When an individual has a cold or an upper respiratory infection, he should attempt to pitch his voice higher and talk "above the cold" with *moderate* volume. Speaking above the cold means using the optimal pitch level. Using this technique for patients in therapy who are experiencing a cold, influenza, or an upper respiratory infection, it was found that almost all were able to maintain a functional voice during the illness. All patients are cautioned that when they have a cold following discharge from therapy, they must talk in a higher pitch above the cold. Some authors advise vocal rest or speaking under the cold. Vocal rest has been found to be a detriment, since following vocal rest the pitch is usually lowered. Speaking under a cold also results in a lowered pitch in our experience.

An overview of the vocal habits prior to the cold or infection of many patients experiencing a cold indicates that vocal misuse involving pitch and tone focus had been a long-term pattern. The infection simply increased the extent of the vocal misuse

---

* By permission Paul J. Moses, *The Voice of Neurosis.* New York, Grune and Stratton, 1954.

enough to heighten the negative vocal symptoms so that the patient became more acutely aware of them. Since the low-pitched voice does not have much carrying power, the tendency is to increase the volume which accelerates the deterioration or misuse of the voice. If the volume is not increased, the vocal misuse may continue for a number of years before the negative vocal symptoms become noticeable and chronic. A cold had precipitated the voice problem in 99 or 20 percent of functional misphonic patients and in 79 or 17 percent of organic dysphonic patients. The cold had occurred from a few months to five or ten years before the patient was seen for therapy.

Persistent coughing can at times create or contribute to the onset and development of a voice disorder. Some voice patients date the onset of their voice problem to a persistent cough. They report that the pitch of the voice was lowered and that speaking became an effort. The continued use of the low pitch added to the pharyngeal and laryngeal irritation further activating the coughing spasm. von Leden and Isshiki (1965, p. 625) in studying the cough mention "the deleterious effect of a cough upon the delicate tissues of the larynx."

Bodily fatigue may contribute to vocal misuse, since usually the pitch is lowered and the tone focus is usually within the laryngopharynx. Bodily fatigue may be due to temporary factors, such as lack of sleep, physical exertion, or sexual orgasm, or due to lasting influences, such as prolonged illness or psychological depression. With bodily fatigue, as with the cold, the patient must speak at the optimal pitch level and range and not allow the pitch to drop. The tone focus must remain within the mask or balanced oral and nasal resonance.

PSYCHOLOGICAL CONTRIBUTORY FACTORS TO VOCAL MISUSE AND ABUSE

Personality and Emotion

Personality, emotions, and psychological problems are found to be contributory or primary causes of voice disorders by some writers. This author has also noted that voice disorders, in turn, may create psychological problems or personality effect.

The degree of the effect depends upon (1) the severity of the problem or how much it interferes with communication; (2) the personality of the individual; (3) the occupation of the individual; (4) the vocal knowledge or extent of voice training the individual has had which in part determines how he will cope with the voice disorder. (This last variable also applies to the amount of effect that emotion has on the voice.)

The three types of social characters according to Riesman with Glazer and Denney (1950) are the inner-directed, the tradition-directed, and the other-directed. Most people in our society appear to be either other-directed or tradition-directed in voice which may create vocal misuse and voice disorders due to the influence of the vocal image, among other factors. The minority who seem to be inner-directed in voice may also become victims of poor vocal knowledge and lack of vocal training. The prognosis in vocal rehabilitation is best for the inner-directed person because he is concerned with his own value system and with what is most rewarding to him.

If the voice problem is severe enough to interfere significantly with communication, personality effect can occur. Most voice patients are talkers, some because of personality need and others because of occupation. One who is in an occupation that requires speaking, such as sales, education, law, or medicine, is more psychologically affected by a voice disorder than is a person who is in a relatively nonspeaking vocation, such as research and accounting.

Emotional and psychological problems may initiate vocal misuse and abuse which lead to voice problems. The same emotional state may create different vocal affects and/or effects in different individuals. For example, anger in some may be shown by an elevated pitch and an increased volume and rate, whereas in others, anger may take the form of a forced low pitch, a deliberate rate, and a limited volume. Also, the same emotional state may cause a different vocal effect in the same individual at different times, depending upon the circumstances and the people involved.

In many patients, the emotions and reactions or tensions are creating the voice problem mainly because the lack of vocal knowledge and of correct vocal usage allows the emotions and tensions to have adverse influence on the voice. Brodnitz (1962, p. 456) agrees: "But there can be no doubt that the lack of technical training makes the voice even more vulnerable to the effects of emotional tensions and anxieties." The well-used voice may reflect feeling states, but it is essentially not controlled by such reactions. Even when the voice is affected, such effect is usually temporary and minimal in the trained voice.

The viewpoint that voice patients are neurotic is maintained by Carrell (1963, p. 260): "While these patients differ greatly one from another, they fit in a greater or lesser degree into the category of the neurotic." Brodnitz (1963, p. 152) concurs:

> Many of the voice patients with functional disorders are highly neurotic persons. The phoniatrist faces the same difficulties that the psychiatrist has to overcome: to surmount the unconscious resistance to any therapy that strikes directly or indirectly at the neurotic dynamics that determine the personality of the patient and, through it, his voice.*

Brodnitz (1958, p. 114) recommends: "A quiet hour spent in discussing the problems of the patient will help much to remove anxieties and restore confident vocal function."

Duncan (1947) notes a relationship between personality and voice disorders. She (p. 167) states:

> Feelings of inferiority among low income groups, and so-called "minority groups," and patterns of family behavior seem to be contributing factors. Closing the valve at the larynx in struggle reaction, a primitive response, results in vocal abuse. Voice often remains an irrational element in behavior. For these cases where these emotional factors seem significant, as they did in at least half of 34 cases of hoarse voice which came under this clinician's instruction, training for insight must be added to exercises.

Duncan suggests that patients with unsatisfactory home adjustment can gain insight through mental hygiene discussions of behavior, problems, topics which create tension, dramatization, and negative practice.

The extreme position regarding personality disturbances caus-

---

* *Archives of Otolaryngology,* 77:152, 1963. Copyright 1963, American Medical Association.

ing voice problems is expressed by Heaver (1958, p. 24) who finds the following descriptive of habitually dysphonic patients:

It is thus apparent that both female and male patients with habitual dysphonia tend to be markedly hostile, sado-masochistic, emotionally immature; they tend also toward paranoid ideation, excessive fantasy and day-dreaming, disorganization of the Ego, withdrawal, and regressive attitudes.

He (pp. 25-26) continues:

The material presented in this study suggests that patients who develop vocal cord abuse resulting in nodes and polyps have been using the voice-box as a natural, biological means of expressing a surcharge of hostile, aggressive impulses. Likewise, they have unconsciously evolved a dysphonic voice production to prevent a breaking through to surface exhibition of these same impulses. Through the dysphonia, the patient is often bailed out of a plaguing dilemma requiring positive decision; the hoarseness interferes with, inhibits, or totally prohibits further verbal communication. Thus, the secondary psychoneurotic gain to the patient is evident; e.g. the avoidance mechanism of hoarseness is socially acceptable. One does not expect verbal participation from another person who cannot talk, be heard, or be understood—or, if that person has been *ordered* by a medical authoritarian figure to be silent.

Bloch (1964) associates voice disorders with psychological problems and he (1962) advises that the physician who treats voice disorders should be aware of the psychological causation. van Thal in Bloch (1962) brings the psychological causation to its fullest fruition by commenting (p. 134): "Not only surgeons but also patients are apt to be satisfied with a 'cured voice.' We must realize that the only justifiable aim is a cured individual." Thus, a voice problem in the eyes of those psychologically and psychiatrically oriented is merely a symptom of an emotionally disturbed and disoriented individual. The removal of the voice disorder itself is not sufficient in their opinion. The entire personality structure must be overhauled, revamped, and rechanneled.

In this author's experience, although patients may have emotional and psychological problems which may affect the speaking voice, most are not consciously aware of misusing the voice. The majority do not have severely disturbed personalities. This author would agree with Goodstein and Murphy. Goodstein (1958, p. 364) comments: "Again it should be clear that much additional research is required and that little is known about personality as an etiological, consequential or therapeutic factor in the disorders of voice." This position is reiterated by Bloch and Goodstein (1971, p. 303): ". . . the number of studies in this area is very few, and little remains known about personality as an etiological, consequential, or therapeutic factor in voice disorders." Murphy (1964, p. 107) writes: "A large number of functional voice disorders are cases of faulty vocal behavior in individuals who do have major personal stresses affecting vocal functioning, but who are essentially normal in terms of general emotional stability."* From clinical observation Murphy's position also appears to be equally valid for benign and premalignant organic voice disorders.

Vocal Image

The vocal image is one of the most vital and determining factors in the creation and continuation of most functional and organic voice disorders (Cooper, 1970n). The vocal image is the sound or voice that the individual either likes or dislikes, either identifies with or disinclines to identify with. Unfortunately, many voice patients have a desire or need to seek voices that assuage their ego rather than meet with their vocal abilities. The vocal image creates counterfeit voices which most individuals find attractive or appealing. Using a counterfeit voice creates vocal misuse and abuse.

Essentially, the vocal image may involve six parameters of the voice. These are the pitch image, the tone focus image, the quality image, the volume image, the breath support or breathing image, and the rate image. The vocal image may exist in discrete form in that an individual may have a vocal image regarding pitch, but not volume, or a vocal image regarding tone focus, but not breath support. Most individuals have a vocal image regarding pitch, tone focus, quality, volume, and breath support. The rate image is found less frequently in voice patients and is less important in the vocal rehabilitative process.

---

* Albert T. Murphy, *Functional Voice Disorders*, p. 107. Copyright 1964, Prentice-Hall, Englewood Cliffs, New Jersey.

There are two types of vocal images: a positive vocal image and a negative vocal image. A positive vocal image is an acceptance of a specific voice type or its various parameters. An individual may have a positive vocal image toward a specific pitch range, a tone focus, a voice quality, a volume level, a type of breath support, or a certain rate. Most individuals have positive vocal images and they are usually directed toward pitch and tone focus. A negative vocal image is the rejection of a type of voice or its parameters. Most negative vocal images relate to pitch, tone focus, quality, volume, and breath support.

Most individuals have both positive and negative vocal images. The emphasis which the individual places upon positive or negative vocal images and the strength of the individual to resist those influences determines the type of vocal image that the individual will acquire and utilize. An individual may have a positive vocal image regarding one vocal aspect, such as a low pitch, and a negative vocal image regarding another aspect, such as nasal voice quality. The formation of a positive vocal image may be based upon a negative vocal image. For example, a negative vocal image regarding a high pitch may lead to a positive vocal image toward a low pitch.

The individual's vocal image is formed essentially by the culture around him, his peer group, his family, and the mass media of communication, namely radio, television, stage, and movies. Unfortunately, a number of individuals in the entertainment field are concerned with a different voice, a saleable voice, not necessarily an efficient or good voice (Cooper, 1970l). These voices are imitated by the general public as well as others in the entertainment field. Lack of vocal knowledge and poor vocal models in all areas of society, including the family, the schools, and the office, all produce the low-pitched voice. The culture or society has created vocal stereotypes, such as the low-pitched, breathy, sexy voice for the female and the low-pitched, rough, masculine voice for the male. The mass media encourages and perpetuates these stereotypes, which, in turn, contribute to the vocal image.

An individual influences others around him to use the type of voice he likes and is in turn influenced by others to use the type of voice they like. For example, a male with a tenor voice may be influenced to use a baritone voice because of negative comments about his squeaky, girlish voice, or because of positive comments about his baritone voice once he lowers his voice. A woman who is told she sounds sexy over the telephone may transfer the lower pitched intimate voice used on the telephone to other situations.

The importance of the body image and its influence upon the vocal image needs exploration and amplification. Clinical practice reveals that patients do relate the two factors or attributes in their own minds and ultimately in their own voices. Some individuals want to sound like they look and others want to sound different from the way they look. A man who looks young may be inclined to gain maturity by lowering the pitch of the voice in order to sound older than he looks. He has a vocal stereotype. He believes that the lower pitch sounds "serious," and that people listen to such a voice and accept the speaker more readily. Another man who is a rugged individual may lower his pitch to sound rugged. For example, an ex-Marine lowered the pitch of voice to fit his body image in reaction to the comment, "Why don't you sound like you look?"

The body image is closely connected to vocal stereotypes. In real life as well as in the mass media, a large or tall man is supposed to have a big, low-pitched voice. A small woman is expected to have a soft, medium or higher pitched voice. Even cartoons depict the toughest, most masculine individual as having a low pitched voice, and the smallest, least impressive individual as having a weak, high pitched voice.

Many patients are playing a vocal role by using a particular voice. Sarbin (1964, p. 188) defines role as "the set of *performances enacted* by the occupant of a status. The extent to which the role enactment corresponds to the expectations held by relevant others is the efficiency, convincingness, or validity of the enactment." Patients may acquire a voice and a vocal image to meet their role commitment.

The vocal image, although occurring frequently and controlling most voice patients, may be absent as a factor in the conscious and perhaps unconscious development of some voices. That is why a few individuals report no vocal image whatsoever as contributing to the onset of their voice disorder; however, in therapy, with the alteration of pitch, tone focus, quality, and/ or volume, an immediate reaction occurs in these patients against the new voice or elements of this voice. For example, if the optimal pitch is different from the habitual pitch, they react sharply and quickly against the new pitch. Van Riper and Irwin (1958) note that the habitual pitch is tied up with the self-concept.

Of the 956 patients seen, 367 or 76 percent of the functional misphonic patients and 368 or 78 percent of the organic dysphonic patients indicated during the initial evaluation that they had a vocal image which influenced the vocal pattern they were using. These patients, as do many other patients, realized immediately that they had a vocal image which had contributed to their voice disorder. Nearly *all* patients, however, realize they have a vocal image when the voice is altered as revealed by their negative comments and reactions to the new voice.

Pitch Image

The strongest positive and negative vocal images revolve around the variable of pitch. Most patients seek a low-pitch level, often stressing the basal or near basal pitch of voice; they have a positive vocal image for a low pitch and a negative vocal image for a high pitch. These individuals are influenced to seek a low pitch by identification of a low pitch with strength, control, assurance, sophistication, knowledgeability, security, relaxation, naturalness, authority, and sexuality. Males are inundated with the concept that the low pitch is masculine; therefore, they are conditioned to be low-pitched. Females identify the low pitch as being sultry and feminine. They attempt to utilize the low pitch of voice because it reflects grace, charm, gentleness, and softness, among the other qualities enumerated.

The need to play a vocal role by many patients is very strong. They want to express the positive qualities they associate with this low-pitch level, because it meets their external and internal personality needs. They are in positions in which they believe that they should reflect immediate and relevant control through their voices. The lawyer meeting with a client is all too often reassuring with his voice, since that is the most apparent and quickly discernible factor to which the client as well as the lawyer responds. The corporate executive reflects control and "coolness" by keeping his pitch steady and often low. Actually the equation of the low pitch to express control is inappropriate since control can easily be expressed in an optimal or natural pitch of voice.

Some patients use the low-pitched voice for negative vocal image purposes in order to mask insecurity and anxiety. They think that the low pitch does not show emotional tensions or anxieties as easily or as clearly as does a higher pitch of voice. A low-pitched voice may be an attempt to mask an accent or an undesirable quality, such as a nasal sound which is repellent or unappealing to the speaker. An individual moving from one section of the country to another may try to conform to the general speech pattern of the new area and finds that lowering the pitch is the easiest way of masking the accent or the voice quality. The ease with which the low pitch can be secured by merely dropping the pitch level to the basal or near basal pitch of voice is one reason why it is so easy to use a low pitch of voice.

Nearly all patients have a negative vocal image for a higher pitch of voice, even though the higher pitch is the optimal pitch, because they usually equate or confuse the higher pitch of voice with a *high* pitched voice. Patients may associate the high pitched voice with insecurity, lack of sophistication, lack of control, lack of virility or sexuality, weakness of personality, effemininity for the male, and a shrill, nagging, or fishmonger sound for the females. The individual must separate his fanciful concepts of voice or vocal stereotypes of a high pitched voice from the real concepts of a natural or optimal pitch of voice.

A major influence upon the use of the low-pitched voice is the mass media of communication which has created a vocal neurosis. Broadcasters in the radio and television industry emphasize the low pitch of voice. Actors and actresses in radio, television, movies, and stage essentially stress the low pitch of voice. Over the years, low-pitched individuals have included Charles Boyer, Humphrey Bogart, Edward G. Robinson, Gregory Peck, Joan Crawford, Tallulah Bankhead, Bette Davis, Marlene Dietrich, and Lauren Bacall. Today, the low pitch is used by many well-known television and motion picture performers. Voices used on radio and television commercials are usually low pitched (Cooper, 1969c).

Actually, the sound of the well-produced or artistic voice of actors and actresses sounds lower than it is, because it utilizes a correct and balanced tone focus. On stage, many knowledgeable performers use a higher pitch of voice in order to project without hurting their vocal folds. In movies they utilize a lower pitch of voice since the microphone is directly above them allowing the electronic media to project the voice.

In all the mass media of communication, the low pitch of voice is stressed by producers and directors, by station managers, and by others who determine who and what will be heard. A pruning process occurs initially for the mass media with the low-pitched voice highly favored and immediately accepted whether correctly or incorrectly produced. For those who have other than a low-pitched voice, in time the vocal image may influence and compel them to use a lower pitch of voice. In essence, the low pitch of voice is an asset in the mass media and an image to strive for when one becomes immersed in the media. Of the many ways mass media voices are misused, pitch is the major variable contributing to that misuse.

Tone Focus and Quality Images

The second and third most important vocal images that prevail among voice patients are those of tone focus and quality. Correct tone focus is balanced oronasolaryngeal resonance in the voice, so that the sound is aesthetic as well as efficient. By aesthetic is meant the quality of voice which appeals rather than rejects. In most instances, a nasal voice in our society would be an unaesthetic voice. A nasal voice has excessive nasopharyngeal resonance or tone focus and may represent uncertainty, insecurity, lack of education, and other similar factors. A hoarse voice may represent the positive aspects, such as control, knowledgeability, sophistication, experience, sexuality, and authority. Although the nasal voice is much more efficient than the hoarse voice, the criterion of patients seen has sharply and concretely favored the hoarse voice as opposed to the nasal voice. Almost all patients have a negative quality image for a nasal voice.

Volume Image

Patients have positive and/or negative images regarding the volume of voice. Some individuals have a positive volume image for a loud voice. Those who are too loud find it purposeful or meaningful since it represents authority, power, strength, control, or other attributes to them.

Most volume images are negative against a loud voice. Patients associate a loud voice with an aggressive, domineering, controlling person. They find a loud voice boisterous, offensive, or impolite, attributes which do not please them. The vocal image in regard to volume may have been established by a negative reaction to a loud, vociferous father, mother, sibling, associate, or friend. Most patients who have a soft voice indicate they resent or are embarrassed by a loud voice.

The most important reaction to a loud voice is the emotional reaction which sets up the aesthetic reaction. A patient who resents or avoids a loud voice usually does so because he associates it with negative personality qualities and equates that loud volume of voice is being unaesthetic. He thereby shifts into a very soft or quiet voice; thus, the vocal image regarding volume is fashioned.

Breath Support Image

There is a positive and negative image regarding breath support. Many patients have a positive image of breath support for speech that directs them to upper chest or clavicular breathing. They are of the view that an expanded chest during inhalation for speech and for vegetative purposes is natural and normal. These individuals believe that upper chest breathing is good for their physical stamina and for their speech. Some male patients have expressed the view that upper chest breathing is manly. Female patients also have indicated that this type of breathing is feminine and sexy.

This image regarding breathing for males and females has been created by grade school teachers and later by physical education teachers. Supposedly, a deep breath is best taken in by expanding the upper torso. As the mythology goes, better speech and healthier bodies are created by upper chest breathing. For the males who have escaped this theory, training in the Armed Services affords them the mythology in full force. Service men are ever keeping their chests expanded for the purpose of better health and fuller voices.

Other patients have a negative image for midsection breath support in that they do not wish a protruding stomach from breathing correctly. Many women express the fear that midsection breathing will cause an enlargement of the diaphragmatic area as well as a large stomach. Many other individuals wear tight clothing around the waist and below so that correct breathing is difficult.

The image regarding breathing has not been reported in the literature nor has it been previously studied in clinical activities. The positive and negative breathing images exist in a number of individuals and have been found to be extremely strong in some individuals.

Rate Image

There are also negative and positive images regarding rate. For example, an individual who speaks quickly may have a positive image regarding a fast rate and/or a negative image regarding a slow rate or vice versa. For those who have a rate image, namely, those who speak too fast or too slowly, this image is based upon poor vocal patterns, poor vocal models, personality traits, mass media, home influences, and environmental pressures. The rate problem is influenced by emotional factors. The individual who speaks too rapidly may do so because he does not want to keep anyone waiting or take too much of their time. He may feel what he has to say is not that important, that he may be presenting incorrect information, or that he may be interrupted before he can conclude the thought. He may be attempting to conceal an articulation problem or an accent.

For many patients experiencing a dysphonia, the rate image is of minor consequence. Most individuals who have a rate problem as well as a dysphonia are speaking too quickly rather than too slowly. Women are more given to a rapid rate than are men. Listeners react more adversely to a rate that is too fast rather than to a rate that is too slow.

The rate image prevails for most situations. A normal and reasonable rate is used for some situations in which the individual is relaxed or comfortable. This applies mainly to individuals with a rapid rate. Individuals using a slow rate rarely change under any conditions. Changing the rate image is basically changing the personality image. This is one of the most difficult aspects to overcome or to alter.

Summary

Almost all voice patients have a vocal image. It is natural and normal to have such an image. Unfortunately, a number of individuals, in order to satisfy a positive vocal image or to avoid a negative vocal image, usurp a voice that is not physiologically natural to their vocal apparatus. They compel that apparatus to conform to their psychological demands and needs without awareness of its ill effects upon the vocal mechanism. The vocal image is a long-term habit supported by vocal myths, vocal stereotypes, and the vocal culture.

The patient with a strong, inept vocal image depicts a *vocal neurosis*, not a general neurosis. A vocal neurosis does not completely incapacitate the individual in communication, but it makes fluidity of communication trying. The vocal neurosis can develop a severe functional voice disorder and eventuate into a severe organic voice problem.

Voice Types

The vocal image voice has specific voice types or variations upon its essential theme. Examples are the second or put-on voice, the intimate or confidential voice, the telephone voice, the sexy or bedroom voice, and the authoritarian voice.

All of these voice types may be used consciously or unconsciously by the speaker. If the voice is consciously manipulated, the individual may pursue this voice for one or more of the following reasons: (1) it sounds resonant and appealing to him; (2) it feels natural or relaxing to him; (3) others have com-

mented favorably upon it; (4) it appears to afford greater listenability and control; and (5) it fulfills an image role and vocal identity by sounding like the type of voice a person in his
position or of his age should have.

If a voice type is unconsciously acquired, it may be for these
following reasons: (1) the individual has unconsciously imitated the voice of a friend or, more often, of a family member;
(2) a cold or illness may initiate a voice type which remains after the cold or illness passes; (3) a personality need or fulfillment may reveal itself through the voice, such as a shy person
using a very quiet volume or an insecure person using a loud
voice of authority to appear secure.

Second Voice or Put-on Voice

The second or put-on voice is an artificial voice in pitch, tone
focus, quality, volume, or rate. This put-on voice may be used
briefly for a temporary situation, used repeatedly in a given situation or with a given person or persons, or used permanently in
all situations. Essentially, there are two types of put-on voices.
One type occurs when the individual switches his voice from
one situation to another, knowingly and purposely, for the effect
it has upon the listeners. The other type of put-on voice is of
a more permanent nature. The individual has acquired a voice
type, such as the voice of authority, the sexy voice, or the confidential voice, and uses that voice as the routine speaking voice.

Intimate or Confidential Voice

Many voice patients selectively use the intimate or confidential voice. This type of voice almost inevitably results in use of
the basal or near basal pitch of voice, often with a minimal
amount of volume. The tone itself may be labeled as exuding
confidence, which gives this voice the term confidential voice.
This type of voice also gives the impression of intimacy, so that
it may also be called the intimate voice. It is a generally accepted and recognized voice type. Some individuals have more need
of it and use it more frequently than others.

The intimate or confidential voice affords many positive qualities to the speaker as well as to the listener. It represents con-

trol, sophistication, culture, knowledgeability, comfort, relaxation, authority, and closeness, among other positive qualities. This type of voice affords affect; it says, "Listen, I have something for your ear alone, and what I have to say is important." Other positive aspects include reduction of a negative tonal quality, such as nasality (or presumed nasality), modification of an accent or an articulation problem, and a soothing sound or manner which calms or quiets the listener, especially if the comments are critical or negative. This voice type attempts to represent a sureness of personality.

The many negative aspects in the use of the intimate voice include a lack of carrying power, a lack of intelligibility, and a lack of flexibility. Listeners complain that they cannot understand what is being said, and individuals who use this voice are often asked to repeat themselves, even when there is a minimal amount of noise during speech.

The intimate or confidential voice is accepted by society and pursued by many as a good voice. Everyone at one time or another uses this voice. Professionals of all fields use it. Doctors use it as part of the "bedside manner" approach. Lawyers use it to be reassuring and knowledgeable. Executives use it as they discuss business deals with associates. Telephone operators, telephone salesmen, disc jockeys, and broadcasting personalities often use the intimate voice.

The majority of those using the intimate or confidential voice do so without much knowledge or awareness of the long-term consequences to their voice. They feel that this voice is the right style and role for them and that it is accepted as being right in the situations in which it is used. An occasional or discreet use of the intimate voice is acceptable as well as reasonable for situations such as brief telephone usage, confidential business meetings, or one-to-one conferences. Unfortunately, this voice, which is initially specific to a given situation, becomes progressively used in more and more situations until it becomes the habitual voice.

The usual auditory and sensory symptoms of a voice disorder may be noted following brief or chronic use of this voice type. Routine use of this type of voice can well affect the vocal folds since the basal or near basal pitch of voice is used frequently. Tension of the laryngeal and pharyngeal musculature is reported by those who seek voice therapy after continued or daily use of this type of voice. This voice type can well be a prelude to an organic dysphonia. It certainly does represent a functional misphonia.

Telephone Voice

The telephone voice has two prominent types. One voice type is the confidential or intimate voice; the other is a loud or vociferous voice. The confidential type of telephone voice affords an intimate quality with the emphasis being on the fact that the individual does not want to be overheard. Generally, those who use this telephone voice type are prone to the same vocal disabilities as those using the confidential voice. In essence, this telephone voice is the confidential or intimate voice transferred to the electronic medium. Many unsophisticated telephone users hearing the so-called sophisticated telephone voice emulate it and eventually fall victim to the vocal disabilities inherent in it. Individuals who use the telephone voice type have a strong positive and negative vocal image regarding the use of this instrument and the voice type applicable to the instrument. Loud and vociferous voices alienate them and so they attempt to avoid a loud voice. Unfortunately, in the process of containing their own volume, they drop to the basal or near basal pitch of the vocal range. As with the confidential voice, sporadic use of this telephone voice type is normal, but too often this voice type is carried over from the telephone to many other speaking situations.

The other type of telephone voice, the loud or vociferous voice, is also widely used. Some who do not normally use this type of voice on the telephone may do so when calling long distance. This voice type may utilize too high or too low a pitch level, too much laryngopharyngeal resonance, and excessive volume. Fortunately, this voice type is not utilized too often and does not appear to be transferred from the telephone to other speaking situations as does the confidential type of telephone voice.

The loud voice may be actuated by the speaker phone. The speaker phone may not pick up a quiet voice which may force the speaker to speak louder with either too high or too low a pitch and laryngopharyngeal tone focus. In point of fact, the speaker phone is one of the most destructive devices causing or contributing to vocal misuse and abuse.

Sexy or Bedroom Voice

The incorporation of sex into the speaking voice is a reality. Men and women attempt and all too frequently succeed in establishing a voice which to the respective user represents masculinity or femininity. This voice may be called the sexy or bedroom voice. It is almost invariably a synthetic or counterfeit voice acquired and used with conscious purpose. This voice often fulfills a need, a want, or a desire on the part of the speaker to represent himself or herself in a given way, namely, sexually or bespeaking of sexuality.

The sexy voice is one of the most pronounced manifestations of the vocal image. It is a very contagious and virulent image, especially since it is encouraged and utilized by a large number of the performing members in the mass media. The sexy voice is preempted at times from adulated movie and television stars, or it may originate from important family members, friends, and associates. If a list were to be mustered of the ten most sexy male voices and the ten most sexy female voices of our decade and then of previous decades, it should prove stimulating to note the patterns of voice appreciated and valued by the public.

The individuals who use the sexy voice have a stereotype of what a sexy voice is and is supposed to be. The voice when broken into its component aspects, such as pitch, quality, tone, and volume, reflects itself in a limited volume, poor and effortful carrying power, a hoarse, husky, breathy tone, and a pitch level which is bordering upon a low monotone. To achieve the so-called sexy voice, the speaker almost invariably drops the pitch below optimal to the basal pitch range, places the tone focus in the lower throat, and possibly incorporates a breathy quality. This pitch level and tone focus create laryngeal and pharyngeal tension when such a voice is maintained.

Because of the ease and swiftness with which the sexy voice can be obtained, this voice is destined to ascend to larger numbers and wider circles. The sexy voice is an established voice, and with continued use, more voice disorders can be expected to develop.

Authoritarian Voice

Those in professions such as law, medicine, engineering, and education, and those in positions of authority, such as executives and administrators, may develop and usurp a voice of authority to match their position as well as to fulfill their internal demands and needs. The voice of authority is a role voice, conceived by those who must display authority in one form or another. This voice not only reflects the speaker's stereotype of what authority sounds like and represents but also conforms to the stereotype of authority from the point of view of the listener. Moses (1954, p. 43) writes: "Authority speaks low. The male teacher, lawyer, judge, and preacher often use a low voice to express authority, utilizing the deepest part of their potential range."*

Sporadic or discreet use of the voice of authority is natural and relevant, as such use is essential for some people in some specific situations. In general, however, the voice of authority is without point or purpose, since the position of the speaker, who is almost invariably a professional in some field of authority, is sufficient cause to have his words and content heard for what they are. Namely, the lawyer is a lawyer who knows law, as is the engineer who knows engineering. The individual using the authoritarian voice is of the view that he needs more than the authority of his position. He feels and believes that his position is not truly representative of him if he does not use this voice type.

The voice of authority may well begin as a voice for specific purposes, specific people, and given circumstances. In time, this voice is transferred to more people and additional circumstances until it becomes not a second voice or put-on voice but the nor-

* By permission Paul J. Moses, *The Voice of Neurosis*. New York, Grune and Stratton, 1954.

mal, routine, and established voice. This voice is productive of laryngeal and pharyngeal tensions. It almost invariably constricts the pitch level to the basal or near basal pitch level and requires additional volume to be heard because the forced low-pitched voice does not carry well or easily. If this voice has been evolved out of purpose and design rather than out of misconception of how to use the voice, it is challenging to alter in vocal rehabilitation, especially if the voice type is firmly and habitually employed.

Summary

In conclusion, all voice types in one fashion or another represent to the individual a commitment to the cultural norms of the society and/or to the stereotypes the individual has regarding the voice for a given person, position, and situation. A voice type, regardless of how created, affords a variety of satisfactions to its respective user. The voice type is usually continued until the negative vocal disabilities are extensive enough to activate concern and consideration for the voice itself by the individual through medical assistance and vocal rehabilitation.

Voice types require variable approaches of vocal rehabilitation. Some require emphasis upon vocal psychotherapy, brief or extended, while other voice types require emphasis upon the mechanics of vocal rehabilitation. Nearly all voice types require vocal psychotherapy, and all require a retraining in the process of correct vocal use. The degree and extent of emphasis in vocal rehabilitation of the mechanical process and of vocal psychotherapy and/or psychotherapy remain for the therapist to determine for each individual patient.

Intra-family Dysphonias

Intra-family dysphonias are defined as two or more members of an immediate family, such as a parent and a child or children, two or more siblings, or both parents, having functional or organic dysphonias. Cornut and Venet (1966) find that 19 mothers and five fathers of 50 dysphonic children were also dysphonic.

Intra-family dysphonias are usually types of positive vocal

images held by one member of a family who identifies with and attempts to imitate the voice of another member. The child's dysphonia is usually created from imitation of the parent's dysphonia. The child may imitate an incorrect pitch level, an improper tone focus, excessive volume, or poor quality. The child may also follow an example of poor vocal hygiene set by the parent, such as yelling and competing with continuous loud noise (television and record players). Intra-family dysphonias may be types of negative vocal images in that one family member attempts to avoid using a voice which is similar to the voice of another family member. This may occur between two siblings. By attempting to avoid a voice type, the child may develop a dysphonia from forcing his voice into inept vocal patterns.

From this author's clinical experience, intra-family dysphonias have been noted in 44 family groups involving 98 individuals.

Number of family groups in which the individuals all had the same dysphonia:
     Nodules (4 family groups).
     Polyps or polypoid degeneration (2 family groups).
     Contact ulcers (1 family group).
     Functional misphonia (17 family groups).
Number of family groups in which the individuals had two or more dysphonias:
     Nodules and functional misphonia (9 family groups).
     Polyps or polypoid degeneration and functional misphonia (2 family groups).
     Contact ulcers and functional misphonia (1 family group).
     Hysterical aphonia and functional misphonia (1 family group).
     Incipient spastic dysphonia and functional misphonia (1 family group).
     Contact ulcers and nodules (1 family group).
     Contact ulcers and polyps (1 family group).
     Nodules and polypoid degeneration (1 family group).
     Polyps and falsetto (1 family group).
     Nodules and paresis and functional misphonia (1 family group).

The most frequent voice problems resulting from intra-family dysphonias are functional misphonia, nodules, and polyps. Although it would be appropriate to treat both (or all) family members in therapy, experience reveals that usually only the one who comes to therapy originally is treated.

Intra-family dysphonias do not occur when a child creates a voice problem by attempting to imitate a parent's voice which is correct for the parent (no dysphonia) but which is not correct for the child. Since the parent in this case does not have a voice problem, the problem is simply one of a vocal image in the child.

PART 2

VOCAL REHABILITATION: DESCRIPTION OF THERAPY

APPROACHES TO THE TREATMENT OF DYSPHONIAS

The five major approaches to treating a dysphonia are surgery, palliative measures, psychological approaches, traditional vocal rehabilitation, and modern vocal rehabilitation which incorporates vocal psychotherapy. The type of treatment pursued for a voice disorder depends upon the philosophy and training of the person treating the patient and his belief as to the etiology of the disorder.

Surgery treats only organic dysphonias. The other four approaches treat both functional and organic dysphonias. The majority of patients with organic dysphonias are treated by surgical procedures; the majority of patients with functional dysphonias are treated by palliative measures. Those physicians using either surgery and/or palliative measures believe the dysphonia may be alleviated or eliminated by medical treatment alone.

Surgery involves the removal of growth(s) from the vocal fold(s) or the injection of synthetic material into a paralyzed vocal fold. Surgery is used to contain malignancies by removing either a portion of the larynx or the complete larynx. Palliative treatment includes vocal rest or vocal silence, antibiotics, gargles, sprays, lozenges, steam, vaporizers, pills, shots, medications, job change, vacation and/or bed rest. Psychological approaches include nondirective psychotherapy, direct psychotherapy, psychoanalysis, and hypnosis. Traditional vocal rehabilitation includes both direct and indirect approaches. The approach which is used by this author is modern direct vocal rehabilitation with vocal psychotherapy, associate therapy, illustrative therapy, and bibliotherapy.

SURGERY

Organic dysphonias which involve benign or premalignant lesions on the vocal folds may be treated by surgery alone, surgery followed by vocal rehabilitation, or vocal rehabilitation alone. Vocal rehabilitation may also be used following the removal of malignant growths on the vocal folds.

Some laryngologists prefer to use surgery alone for the removal of growths on the vocal folds. However, a review of voice patients indicates that repeated surgical procedures are being performed due to the return of growths. This recurrence is essentially due to vocal misuse and abuse.

Laryngologists should be aware of the possible need for vocal rehabilitation following surgery which removed a growth(s) from the vocal folds. The removal of tissue from the vocal folds should be the beginning of a vocal recovery. All too often the surgery is the entire assistance for the patient.

Brodnitz (1958, p. 113), a laryngologist, discusses the relationship between surgery and vocal rehabilitation.

> Surgical removal is necessary in the majority of benign lesions of the cords. But in small lesions of relatively recent standing, such as small nodules, thickening of the cords, small contact ulcers without pronounced granulation, vocal therapy alone may effect a disappearance of tissue changes together with the restoration of a normal voice.
>
> On the other hand, larger and solidified nodules, well-defined polyps, general polypoid thickenings of the cords, and contact ulcers with extensive granulation require surgical intervention, to be followed by vocal rehabilitation. Without such vocal retraining recurrences are frequent since the underlying cause of the lesion continues to be effective.

Kleinsasser (1968, p. 41) makes the following recommendations:

> Speech therapy is always indicated after the removal of nodules or contact pachydermia, and sometimes after decortications or removal of polyps and papillomas. Speech therapy will be necessary particularly if the patient develops a voice pitch that is too deep or too high, or if he phonates with the false vocal cords.

In discussing contact ulcer of the larynx, Cooper and Nahum (1967, p. 42) write:

> The surgeon must always keep in mind that any surgical procedure for this disease has only temporal value and does not alter the basic etiologic factors which are operating and which will continue to operate. Without concomitant vocal therapy, surgery alone will usually fail to correct the problem and may aggravate and accelerate the disease process.*

---

* *Archives of Otolaryngology*, 85:42, 1967. Copyright 1967, American Medical Association.

Vocal rehabilitation following a surgical procedure is for two purposes: (1) to eliminate vocal misuse and abuse in order to prevent the recurrence of the growth, and (2) to restore an efficient voice to the patient. A surgical procedure does not remove nor alter poor vocal patterns and vocal misuse and abuse which have produced and will continue to produce an inefficient and pathological voice.

Prior to surgery, the patient should be made aware that the postsurgical voice may be worse than the presurgical one and may require vocal rehabilitation, even though the surgery is successful insofar as removal of the growth is concerned. Personality effect and severe mental trauma may well occur if the patient is not prepared for the possibility of a poor voice and of the need for vocal rehabilitation. Unless patients are cautioned, they are under the assumption that the surgery will remove their problem and that the growth(s), if it does return, will not recur for many years.

Other patients wait for their old (pregrowth) voice to return following a surgery. A patient may become disturbed after waiting months or even years for his voice to return only to realize he is in need of voice therapy. Additionally, there is the problem of the patient whose old voice returns following surgery, but he is unaware that this voice is productive of the growth. With continued use of this old voice he may once again require surgery, since the old voice pattern is programmed for vocal misuse and abuse.

Following a surgical procedure, the pitch of voice may be quite unstable. The optimal pitch must be located and stabilized in vocal rehabilitation. Vocal therapy also includes establishment of the proper tone focus, reasonable volume, and correct breath support. These and other necessary changes are described fully later in this chapter. Vocal rehabilitation may be necessary following surgery for the injection of a synthetic substance, such as silicone or Teflon, into a paralyzed vocal fold (see Paralytic Dysphonia).

This author's experience supports vocal rehabilitation with vocal psychotherapy (fifth method), either alone or following surgery, depending upon the discretion of the laryngologist who determines the practicality or relevance of surgery. Although

Peacher (1961) found that surgery prolonged the vocal rehabilitative process in a follow-up of 70 contact ulcer patients, my clinical experience with 470 organic dysphonic patients indicates
that the surgical procedure may be a motivating factor which
activates the patient to enter vocal rehabilitation. Of the 180
postoperative patients seen (no lesion present, one or more surgeries) and of the 66 postoperative and return patients seen (lesion present, one or more surgeries), 75 percent of the postoperative patients and 74.4 percent of the postoperative and return patients entered therapy. Of those entering therapy, 91.1
percent postoperative and 89.8 percent postoperative and return
patients completed therapy. Of the 224 patients seen in the no
surgery group, 70.5 percent entered therapy and 93.7 percent
completed therapy. In comparing therapy results for the groups,
excellent results were achieved by 65 percent of the postoperative patients, by 79.5 percent of the postoperative and return patients, and by 73.6 percent of the no surgery patients. Interest-
ingly, of the postoperative patients, only 25.6 percent had had
two or more surgeries, but of the postoperative and return patients, 53 percent had had two or more surgeries. These statistics
indicate the best results for the group having the most surgeries
(postoperative and return), followed by the no surgery group,
and last of all by the postoperative group. Repeated surgeries apparently help motivate the patient. (See Results for charts and
further discussion.)

PALLIATIVE TREATMENT

Most functional dysphonic patients are afforded palliative
measures to deal with their voice problems. Frequently patients
have been given antibiotics (injections and medication) for
many months in order to resolve a voice disorder. This method
of treatment is utilized by a number of laryngologists who remain unaware that the inflammation of the vocal folds may be
due to misuse of voice rather than to viruses, allergies, and infections. Tarneaud, a well-known laryngologist (1958, p. 10),
writes:

> Many a physician throughout the world pretends to be a voice
> specialist. To all their patients, whatever the affection involved, they

apply the same treatment: intra-laryngeal oil injections, daubing of the vocal cords, ionisation or faradisation of the larynx, . . . When the patients feel preoccupied, uneasy, anxious, obsessed, as some singers do, the treatment then is but disguised psycho-therapy, but it is unable to restore the correct coordinations and synergies of the speaker's or singer's voice. Consequently, orators and singers thus treated for months and years just give up because they never recover their vocal possibilities.

Antibiotics are entirely relevant and within the medical jurisdiction for colds or infections that are creating voice disorders. Unfortunately, antibiotics have essentially no basis or relevance for voice disorders that are created by vocal misuse and abuse. Antibiotics also have no purpose in the resolution of voice disorders that continue following the end of a cold or infection. The postcold or postinfection voice problem occurs in approximately 15 to 20 percent of all voice disorders.

Vocal rest or vocal silence is another of the leading prescriptive remedies afforded voice patients. Medical personnel as well as lay persons often prescribe vocal rest. The presumptive belief for this approach is (1) that the vocal folds tire from natural use rather than from misuse and abuse, and (2) that vocal rest will revitalize the tired vocal folds so that a clear and easy voice is produced.

Vocal rest is essentially irrelevant to most voice disorders when and if these disorders are caused by vocal misuse. Vocal rest is misleading to the patient and may become a hindrance because (1) it does not allow the patient to realize he is misusing his voice, since following variable periods of vocal rest, the voice usually returns; and (2) following the vocal return, the voice is again misused, and further vocal rest is necessary. The need for repeated instances of vocal rest reveals the extent and severity of progressive vocal misuse and/or abuse.

Vocal rest is freely prescribed but is seldom observed by those it is intended to assist. Personality effect is sharp and immediate to vocal rest, and few patients are able to fulfill the dictum: "Be silent for a week or two," or "Rest your voice for a couple of weeks." Nearly all patients afforded vocal rest have reported that they essentially failed to observe it, except following a surgical procedure and even then vocal rest was not complete. Vocal rest is usually a mythical panacea.

Vocal rest may be relevant following a surgical procedure upon the vocal folds and would then be applicable for a week or two. Longer periods of vocal rest following surgery can create vocal problems in causing a weakness of unused laryngeal muscles. Some physicians also advise vocal rest for a week or so prior to surgery so that the area is not as inflamed and the growth is more clearly defined. Other times when vocal rest is appropriate are during severe illnesses or after bouts of yelling, when the vocal folds may be inflamed and possibly thickened. Vocal rest will assist in the normalization of the return of the routine voice. Once the routine voice is back, vocal rest is no longer applicable.

In some rare instances vocal rest may be used at the beginning of vocal therapy if the voice is so hoarse that the optimal pitch cannot be determined. This one- to two-week period of vocal rest is necessary for only a fraction of perhaps 1 percent of all voice patients. Although it is an extremely infrequent procedure, voice specialists might find it helpful at some time or another.

Whispering is sometimes recommended following surgery. Differentiation should be made between a true whisper and a forced whisper.

The true whisper is appropriate as a temporary method for permitting the patient who has had surgery on the vocal folds a form of communication which enables him to meet business and personal demands and commitments. In the true whisper, the vocal folds do not approximate and there is no tenseness nor effort in its production. Since the true whisper has no carrying power, it can be used only for interpersonal communication in quiet surroundings. Postsurgical voice patients have not encountered any vocal or medical problems when the true whisper is utilized only for a brief period of time following the surgery.

The forced or stage whisper does have a moderate degree of carrying power, but its production not only creates extreme vocal fold tensions, but also requires a great amount of physical effort. Since the mechanism of the forced whisper is abusive to the recuperating vocal folds, this type of whisper must be avoided, especially during the postoperative period.

Other palliative measures, such as gargles, sprays, lozenges, vaporizers, and steam are also essentially irrelevant insofar as voice disorders are concerned. These measures have a slight purpose only in easing laryngeal and pharyngeal pain created by vocal misuse and abuse. They soothe the inflamed area for a short period of time. Some symptoms, such as hoarseness, may disappear briefly, but they will usually persist despite palliative treatment. These palliatives merely assuage or mask the pain or irritation in the throat, thereby addicting the patient to repeated doses without eliminating the causative factors and enabling the patient to continue using and misusing the voice. Many a voice patient reports a long history of utilizing these palliative measures, with the essential problem of vocal misuse and its attendant laryngeal and pharyngeal discomfort increasing progressively.

As a concomitant for vocal rehabilitation, in the early stages of therapy, one or more of these palliative measures for symptom containment and relief may make the patient feel more comfortable and amenable to therapy; however, these measures used in isolation are useless in the containment and elimination of the voice disorder. Nearly all voice patients are able to abstain from these palliative measures once they are made aware of the cause and effect of the symptoms of voice misuse.

Job change or change of occupation is a prescriptive recommendation afforded the voice patient all too often by unsophisticated medical practitioners and supervisory personnel. For those prescribing such an occupation change the underlying belief is that experiencing vocal fatigue is natural to some and indicative of inherent vocal weakness either of the larynx or of the physical condition of the patient. Occupations that require little or minimal speaking are recommended for these individuals who experience negative voice symptoms. What is really needed is a voice change, not a job change.

Unfortunately, far too many individuals heed the dictum of job change and become vocal hermits. One patient remained at home, seldom answering the telephone, because she was advised that continued vocal rest was the only answer to her voice problem. She no longer assisted her husband in the store and the personality effect was severe. Another patient gave up a lecturing career and became a researcher because he was advised to use his voice minimally to avoid vocal fatigue.

Vacation and bed rest are two other palliative measures that are subscribed to as a method to meet voice disorders. Those prescribing such measures presume that the patient is mentally or physically fatigued and in need of rest or an environmental change. The inadequacy of these measures is proven time and time again as these patients reexperience the vocal symptoms and voice disorder once they return to normal activity. Some are not free of the vocal symptoms even during the rest or vacation. The pressure of the environment may not be the basic cause of these voice symptoms. Temporary vocal effect from tensions is experienced by most, but the effect need not be lasting if the patient has vocal knowledge and ability in correct vocal usage.

Patients should not be asked to change their personality because of vocal misuse. If a patient is outgoing and dynamic, he should not be told to speak less or to be quiet in order to save his voice. Containment of the personality is not only unrealistic, but it is also unfair to the patient. Patients also should not be told simply to speak in a relaxed manner, since what usually happens is that the patient drops the pitch to the basal level, uses little volume, and in the process further misuses the voice.

Regarding palliative measures, Guthrie (1940) reports that local treatments are secondary and subsidiary to orthophonic or reeducative methods. Not atypical is the patient with functional misphonia who was given twenty-five different medications, including Librium®, sulfa, Polycillin®, tetracycline, atrophine, and ACTH as well as ultrasonic medcolator treatments for hoarseness and laryngitis over a period of years by two laryngologists. The patient in this case was markedly hoarse and had secured no relief from the administration of such medication over this protracted period of time. This patient's functional misphonia was eliminated by vocal rehabilitation. Douglas (1950, p. 383), a medical specialist, writes:

> The patient is alarmingly frequent who has been treated for hoarseness supposedly due to sinusitis, deviated nasal septum, enlarged palatine tonsils, infected or noninfected, for one or two years prior to seeking other medical advice, when his symptoms have ei-

ther failed to have been alleviated or have progressed. Not infrequently, the patient is seen to have a uvulectomy or wholesale dental extractions performed in an attempt to treat the hoarseness or laryngeal sensations.

Tarneaud (1947, p. 14) concurs: "The patients often receive wrongly and unsuccessfully treatment for chronic laryngitis, whereas, only phoniatric treatment—considering the somatic and psychological etiology—is promising."

Palliative measures are not curative measures. They do not eliminate; they merely alleviate. They are misleading to the patient and contributory to the continued voice disorder and personality effect that accrues to a patient with a voice disorder. Palliative measures, nonetheless, continue to be the pervasive measures prescribed by most medical personnel and accepted by most individuals experiencing voice disorders.

PSYCHOLOGICAL APPROACHES

Directive and nondirective psychotherapy and psychiatric treatment have been presented as measures to contain or eliminate voice disorders. The presumptive view for these approaches is that the individual with a voice disorder is consciously or unconsciously misusing his voice as part of a personality or character disorder, as previously discussed. Analysis of the psyche may do wonders for the individual and his personality, but its effect upon the individual's real or potential voice is extremely limited, if not nil. Wolberg (1967, p. 83) writes: "The speech therapist is concerned with modifying speech patterns, the psychotherapist with altering the general personality structure." Those extremely limited cases that have been reported where the individual undergoing psychotherapy or psychiatric treatment have improved the voice or overcome the voice disorder are quite rare. If and when the voice is improved by psychological or psychiatric measures alone, the essential question must be, "What has the voice improved to?" and "Who is doing the judging of the voice?"

In those cases where psychotherapy or analysis have produced new and startling voices from misused or troubled voices, the change from the old to the new voice is recognized by all, but the fact that the new voice does not utilize an optimal pitch range or have an efficiency to it is not recognized. The index utilized by psychotherapists or psychiatrists is highly subjective and superficial. Falsetto voices that change to low-pitched voices are presumed to reflect the excellence of psychological insight and assistance. Altering a voice disorder from one end of the spectrum, such as the high pitch of falsetto, to the other end, such as a bass voice, when the range is really baritone, is merely substituting one voice disorder for another, but to a lesser extent. There is no question that the psychological approach can change voices in specific types of voices, such as falsetto or hysterical aphonia, but even in these types of cases, the end result in voice may eventually result in severe vocal disorders once again for the patient. The new voice disorder may not be as stigmatic, but it may create personality effect that will be as severe; the patient may presume that his neurosis is once again prevailing and that analysis is regressing. He does not consider voice therapy because he is not oriented to direct measures for his voice. He has been led to believe that such measures are superficial to his real problem, a personality disturbance.

Most voice patients who have undergone psychotherapy or psychoanalysis have often remained burdened with voice disorders despite their extended periods of training. The psychotherapists or psychiatrists in these cases have neither concerned themselves with the voice disorder, not recognizing such symptoms as indicating a voice disorder, nor have they been able to adequately prescribe for it. Some psychiatrists and psychotherapists themselves have voice problems or vocal symptoms.

Psychotherapists and psychiatrists are generally unsophisticated in diagnosing voice disorders, what constitutes such, and what measures are necessary to overcome such disorders. Greater insight into one's psyche does not beget a better voice. Catharsis, insight, and personality reintegration may afford more comfort, greater ease, more mental and physical relaxation, as well as more meaningful communicative responses to others and to one's self, but it does not change a pathological voice to a nonpathological voice. The elements of pathological voice are altered only when the individual experiencing such vocal pathology is made aware of the variable elements of voice, such as pitch, volume, tone focus, and breath support, and is taught the correct use of these factors which are then made automatic in spontaneous communication.

Only a few psychotherapists and psychiatrists are cognizant of the variables involved in voice, and especially in vocal pathology. Still fewer are able to deal with these voice variables as part of their practice. Those psychotherapists and psychiatrists who are knowledgeable and trained in voice disorders are most helpful in the resolution of some types of voice disorders.

Weiss and Schick, two psychiatrists, have stated quite explicitly that voice disorders must be dealt with by vocal rehabilitation. Schick (1966, p. 140) writes: "From our long and varied experience we have learned that vocal disturbances are treated far more efficaciously by functional therapy than by psychotherapeutic measures alone." Weiss (1955, p. 215) concurs:

> The voice and the psychological make-up of an individual mutually influence each other. If a person is psychologically disturbed, the voice suffers, and in turn the deterioration of the voice exerts a negative influence upon the psyche. We can approach this vicious circle from either the psychological or the vocal angle. Psychotherapy is often a hazardous and always a lengthy procedure and, as mentioned above, the voice would have to be treated in any case. On the other hand, in the treatment of the voice we feel on pretty firm ground. Attacking the formerly vicious circle from this point, we arrive, by improving the phonation, at influencing the psyche in a favorable manner. This, in turn, creates more favorable conditions for the voice itself. Thus the vicious circle has been converted into a "virtuous" one.

Psychotherapy or psychoanalysis for most voice cases is too time-consuming and too circuitous. Bloch (1959, p. 116) says: "Moses affirms that well-planned vocal psychotherapy is capable of replacing a more extensive type of routine psychotherapy."

Hypnosis is another type of treatment which recently has come into the cynosure of public attention. Hypnosis is an attempt to convince the patient that vocalization is easy. The hypnotist is usually untrained in the variables of voice, and therefore, the net result of hypnosis in voice cases is that the voice may be less effortful and less strained to the untrained ear. To the trained voice therapist, the vocal misuse is merely masked or covered by less volume, but the essential misuse of pitch, quality, tone focus, and inept breath support prevails. Hypnotists, like psychotherapists and psychiatrists, indicate a marked tendency to utilize the basal or near basal pitch of voice. Apparently their own vocal image supports their belief that a low-pitched voice with moderate or light volume reveals personality control, appropriate role identity, and similar positive qualities. Laryngologists as well as general practitioners have not favored hypnosis. Brodnitz (1963) finds that the results of hypnosis regarding voice patients with spastic dysphonia are disappointing. This author would agree. In fact, one patient, using self-hypnosis to improve the voice, developed spastic dysphonia.

In essence, psychotherapy and hypnosis do not apply directly to most voice disorders. In those cases where personality affect needs to be altered and where the personality problem is the essential problem, then psychotherapy and psychiatric attention should be the fundamental approach followed by or concurrent with vocal rehabilitation.

Voice disorders have developed and continued often by poor vocal training and inept vocal knowledge. These voice disorders are amenable to direct vocal rehabilitation and *vocal* psychotherapy. Nearly all voice patients either report a vocal image as contributing to the onset and development of the voice disorder or realize the extent of the influence of the vocal image upon their voice once a new voice is being reestablished for them. The vocal image is socially and culturally developed, and it requires direct vocal psychotherapy to define and detail to the patient the development of such an image.

TRADITIONAL VOCAL REHABILITATION

Traditional vocal rehabilitation concerns itself with the variables of voice: pitch, tone focus, quality, volume, breath support, and rate. The traditional approach treats the vocal variables first in isolation and then in combination. An excellent discussion of the traditional approach is found in Anderson (1961). Traditional vocal rehabilitation includes both direct (Anderson) and indirect (Froeschels) methods for locating the optimal pitch level.

Although this author treats these six variables, he differs in the sequential treatment of the variables, the emphasis upon certain variables, and the techniques used for correcting these variables. His concepts and techniques will be discussed under each variable. Since this author stresses the concept that optimal pitch is the most important variable dealt with in modern vocal rehabilitation, and because the approach and the emphasis on pitch in modern vocal rehabilitation are so different from the traditional approach, the factor of pitch will be discussed in detail for a more complete understanding of the two approaches.

Optimal pitch level and range is a concept that is recognized and noted by many, including Anderson (1961), West, Ansberry and Carr (1957), Van Riper and Irwin (1958), Fairbanks (1960) (natural pitch), Williamson (1945), Peacher (1966), Flower (1959), and Greene (1964). Pronovost (1942) and Snidecor (1943, 1951) have studied the pitch of superior speakers. Pronovost (1942) has outlined the various mechanical methods to directly locate the optimal or natural pitch level. An indirect method of locating this pitch has been presented by Weiss and Beebe (1950).

There are those few who disavow the existence of the optimal pitch and/or its relationship to voice disorders. It can be unequivocally stated from clinical experience of over 1400 voice cases that not only does the optimal pitch concept exist, but also the lack of such a pitch level is responsible for nearly all voice disorders.

Direct Approach

The neophyte voice therapist may initially utilize one or more of the mechanistic approaches outlined by Provonost (1942) as a tentative means of approximating the optimal pitch level until his ear is refined to the degree that these approaches are not necessary. The reasons for possible failure of the mechanistic approach are as follows:

1. Few individuals understand or are fully trained in its methodology. Clinical voice experience in a training institution tends to be haphazardly presented and inefficiently rendered. Few qualified voice therapists (those with clinical experience with several hundred voice patients) exist on faculty staffs. Still fewer of those qualified have the time to personally supervise students who require careful training in this highly technical area.

2. Many of these methods, especially those most recommended, are based on the lowest sustained pitch or basal pitch. Cooper and Yanigahara (1971) in studying the basal pitch level show that the basal pitch level varies one to three semitones throughout the day and from day to day. If the basal pitch is utilized in establishing the optimal pitch, then the optimal pitch could differ at varying times throughout the day and from day to day.

3. Mistaken identity of the vocal fry for the basal pitch would also alter the location of the correct optimal pitch.

4. Voice therapists may not have a trained musical ear, so they are unable to establish the basal pitch per se and relate the basal pitch to the piano.

5. Average or normal speakers often have a limited pitch range. Any method which uses the total pitch range, or a certain number of notes from the bottom of the pitch range, may have the individual speaking at the top of his pitch range or at too high a level.

6. The dysphonic patient may not have the ability to sing or hum up and down the scale in order to allow for the delineation of the entire pitch range.

The emphasis upon the location of the optimal pitch is appropriate, but the methods used to establish optimal pitch level and range are too mechanistic, too tentative, and too approximate. After describing one method of locating the optimal pitch, Anderson (1961, p. 85) writes: "Experiment with the new-found pitch by singing various vowel sounds on that level and chanting on a monotone. Proceed above and below it to discover whether an adjacent pitch might not give better results, since the method just described is not absolute but only approximate." Unfortunately, students who pursue this approach may not take Anderson's suggestion and may rely too heavily or entirely upon the accuracy of the mechanistic, objective approach without tempering it with a fine, subjective ear.

Indirect Approach

A major indirect traditional approach is the chewing method advocated by Froeschels, Weiss, and Brodnitz. In this method, the patient eliminates hyper- and hypofunction from the voice through exercises, one of which is vocalization while chewing. The patient is advised to chew naturally and at the same time produce sound. This sound is assumed to be at the proper pitch level. Weiss and Beebe (1950) have compiled a series of articles that discuss the chewing method. Cooper (1971c, p. 597) describes advantages and disadvantages of this method in some detail:

> The method appears to be effective basically in the hands of those who are familiar with its purposes and its limitations, and who are also knowledgeable in vocal rehabilitation. However, the recommendation that the chewing method is *the* method is without foundation. This method affords many limitations in actual practice aside from all theoretical considerations. The optimal pitch level and range are given neither by the therapist nor requested of the patient. The new pitch that is afforded the patient via the chewing method may well create extended or extensive hyper- and/or hypofunction of the voice. The chewing method is indirect or non-direct and places the responsibility on the patient who must determine which pitch range or level feels comfortable. (The traditional approach is directive in that the optimal pitch level and range are afforded the patient.) Nondirective vocal rehabilitation is highly dangerous in that it allows a patient to become his own therapist and thereby presumes that vocal assistance can be rendered by a basically non-assistant therapist. In actuality, experience has shown that the optimal pitch level and range are uncomfortable for many at first since the vocal muscles are being realigned. The discomfort quickly disappears as the optimal pitch level is utilized. However, the patient would not originally choose this range as comfortable, functional, satisfactory, or aesthetically appealing. In addition, the chewing approach is concerned with neither a development or extension of range nor with the aesthetic element of voice—namely, the tone.

Other limitations are (1) the patient can chew and produce sound at the incorrect pitch level as easily as he can at the correct pitch level, and (2) the patient may object to chewing and producing sound. Froeschels (1943, p. 129) himself makes this very point: "Many persons never get entirely used to it, but they can learn to maintain the idea of chewing while they are thinking of what they are saying."

Regarding the chewing method, Van Riper and Irwin (1958, pp. 293-294), although they admit "lack of intensive training in the technique," have found "marked resistance in many patients" who "complain about the abnormality of the obvious movements." They continue:

> And we also find that, although the patient is able to produce better pitch levels and better quality while working with *us*, the improvement is often merely temporary. The necessity for constantly thinking of chewing evidently becomes burdensome to the case and it distracts him from the self-hearing of the new voice which is so important in stabilizing it. We also find the transition from overt chewing to "mental chewing" is not accomplished easily. [*]

They do note success with a few younger cases.

There are other approaches that may be included as nondirect. Laguaite and Waldrop (1964, p. 190) summarize: "Therapy designed to teach a patient to phonate in an easy, relaxed manner should restore the voice to its 'optimum' pitch without the use of special techniques." In this author's experiences, relaxed phonation without direction often results in use of a basal or near basal pitch level. Shearer (1959), in following the cybernetic theory, has the patient record his voice at many different pitch levels and qualities. The patient is asked to select the most pleasing pitches and qualities. He (p. 281) continues:

> Soon the patient becomes proficient at speaking in different voices and indicates that he no longer knows which is his "normal" speaking voice. The patient thus begins to modify his own voice in the direction of the optimal pitch level of his own choosing.

This method presumes the patient can judge his own pitch level correctly. These two nondirective approaches do not appear to be feasible for most voice patients.

MODERN VOCAL REHABILITATION WITH VOCAL PSYCHOTHERAPY

Modern vocal rehabilitation differs from the traditional (direct and indirect) approach in that the location of the optimal pitch, although direct, does not depend on mechanistic methods. A natural method is utilized to locate the optimal pitch. The next most important variable is tone focus. Quality and volume

---

[*] Charles Van Riper and John V. Irwin, *Voice and Articulation*, pp. 293-294. Copyright 1958, Prentice-Hall, Englewood Cliffs, New Jersey.

are basically dependent upon pitch and tone focus. Breath support buttresses the four preceding variables. Rate is usually of minor consideration, unless it interferes with the process of vocal rehabilitation.

The traditional viewpoint is that relaxation must precede or accompany vocal rehabilitation. This author finds that general relaxation is not possible until therapy is complete. The process of locating and maintaining the correct pitch, tone focus, quality, volume, and breath support in and of itself is a tensing process. Concentration upon the new process is tensing, just as learning to play a new number on a musical instrument is tensing and tiring. To develop any new motor pattern requires a marked degree of tension. Only when the motor pattern is mastered is the tension reduced and eliminated. At that time general bodily relaxation is possible.

Modern vocal rehabilitation incorporates vocal psychotherapy, a most vital aspect in permanently altering the voice. This approach also uses associate therapy, illustrative therapy, and bibliotherapy.

Modern vocal rehabilitation also utilizes extensive tape replay of the patient's old and new voices. The process of recording and playback with comparative analysis is an important part of vocal therapy.

Pitch and Tone Focus

An incorrect pitch is one of the most important variables in the creation and maintenance of a voice problem or voice disorder. The incorrect pitch almost always creates an incorrect tone focus. When the incorrect pitch is too low, which occurs in the majority of voice disorders, the laryngopharyngeal resonance is almost always emphasized. When the pitch is too high, there may be too much nasopharyngeal resonance. As Holmes (1931, p. 244) explains: "All of the cases which have incorrect 'placement' present pitch levels which are either above or below the normal pitch." In most cases, the location of the optimal pitch level is the key factor in locating the correct tone focus (balanced oronasolaryngopharyngeal resonance).

In modern vocal rehabilitation, the patient is directed to his optimal pitch and proper tone focus by the voice therapist.

Brodnitz (1966a, p. 238) states that the direct manipulation of pitch is a mistake. "Manipulation of pitch is a hazardous undertaking for which no sound objective basis exists, and it is one that depends too much on the subjective preference of the therapist. If general hyperfunction is eliminated from the voice, pitch usually takes care of itself." The manipulation of pitch is not a hazardous undertaking for the competent voice therapist who has the understanding and ability to identify the proper pitch level for a given voice. Manipulation of pitch is a hazardous undertaking only if the therapist lacks training and sophistication in determining the optimal pitch level.

Others do not think the therapist can or should locate the optimal pitch. Gildston and Gildston (1968, p. 124), using speech pathologists and undergraduate speech majors as listeners, summarize:

> The most significant finding was that both sophisticated and naive listeners labeled as optimal a number of pitch levels with a modal difference of almost an octave at the extremes. . . . It was concluded that an individual may select from among several optimal pitch ranges, depending upon personal and cultural preferences.

In this author's opinion, most speech pathologists should not necessarily be considered "sophisticated" listeners in judging the optimal pitch level. This category should include only speech and/or voice therapists with adequate training and several years experience with voice patients. This author would agree that the vast majority of speech pathologists may not be experienced enough to judge optimal pitch and that most individuals choose pitch because of personal and cultural preferences, which is one of the causes of widespread vocal misuse.

Gildston and Gildston (1968, p. 125) are of the view that:

> Not only is it difficult, if not impossible, to determine optimal pitch level initially, but, frequently, the patient's range is so restricted we cannot induce him to produce voice at the level that will eventually be determined to be optimal for him. The first task is often to extend the range of acceptable tone.

Weiss (in Gildston and Gildston, 1968, p. 125) agrees:

> I would like only to emphasize that find [sic] the optimal pitch in

the beginning should not be considered as a basic goal. Often the patient is not able to produce or to reveal his optimal pitch. He needs first a certain therapy and loosening up his manner of phonation before the optimal pitch can be found.

Clinical experience indicates that only 1 percent to 2 percent of over 1400 voice cases were so severely dysphonic that the optimal pitch could not be determined in the initial session. The first task is to locate the optimal pitch level which of itself extends the "range of acceptable tone."

The knowledgeable voice therapist must of necessity make a subjective judgment as to the correct pitch level for the given patient. He must not determine the optimal pitch level according to likes or dislikes which he internally or externally voices. He must be knowledgeable and perceptive enough in realizing what is the optimal pitch level for the patient. Every judgement made by a competent or incompetent voice therapist is a subjective statement. *The subjective evaluation becomes objective when the therapist is able to produce a patient who is free from dysphonia.* Greene (1964, p. 134) believes: "The therapist is generally able to assess the natural pitch from his voice although dysphonic, and should give him the pitch she wishes him to imitate in all phonation exercises."[*]

The optimal pitch level and the correct tone focus must be found as quickly as possible. It can usually be located within a matter of seconds in the initial evaluation. The optimal pitch level and proper tone focus are located at the same time since they are basically interdependent upon one another. In over 90 percent of the patients seen, the pitch needed to be raised and the tone focus transferred from the laryngopharynx to the oronasopharynx for balanced resonance.

In a study by this author (1972) the fundamental frequencies before and after therapy for 155 dysphonic patients in fourteen dysphonias were determined from spectrographs. Following vocal rehabilitation, the fundamental frequencies for 150 patients of the total group of 155 dysphonic patients showed an increase when compared to the fundamental frequencies of these patients

---

[*] M. Greene, *The Voice and Its Disorders,* 2nd ed. London, Pitman Medical Publishing Co., 1964.

prior to vocal rehabilitation; therefore, of 155 patients, 150 were raised in pitch during therapy. The fundamental frequencies or pitch levels varied markedly among patients before therapy. The same was true after therapy, although each patient had achieved his optimal pitch level. As was expected, no standard pitch level was found to exist for individual patients and average pitch levels should not be considered when locating individual optimal pitch levels. Two factors indicate that the pitch located for each patient in this study was that patient's optimal pitch: (1) completion of vocal rehabilitation with a rating of excellent or good, which indicated an alleviation and/or elimination of the dysphonia and of negative vocal symptoms (sensory, auditory, and visual); and (2) the findings of the follow-up that 98% of 128 patients involved in the follow-up had remained excellent or good three months to seven years following the completion of vocal rehabilitation.

A very simple and straightforward method of locating the optimal pitch level has been successfully utilized in over 1400 voice patients in the last ten years. The simplicity of the method in locating the optimal pitch level is what makes it highly utilitarian and pragmatic. The patient is simply asked to say "um-hum" using a rising inflection with the lips closed, as though he were spontaneously and sincerely agreeing with what was just said. It is vital to underscore the fact that this "um-hum" be spontaneous and sincere.

The "um-hum" may be either natural or forced. A natural "um-hum," which is easy and gentle, will be felt around the sides and lower portion of the nose and around the lips. A forced "um-hum" either uses too much volume or is focused within the laryngopharynx. Both the natural and forced "um-hum" will produce vibration about the nose and lips, so the therapist must guide the patient in producing a natural and not a forced "um-hum." The optimal pitch level is clearly evident when the patient follows this procedure in most cases. As Greene (1964, p. 134) describes: "When the optimal pitch is sounded the voice leaps into prominence, being so much more rich and resonant that there is no mistaking its rightness."*

---

* M. Greene, *The Voice and Its Disorders*, 2nd ed. London, Pitman Medical Publishing Co., 1964.

To determine the validity of the clinical tool "um-hum" as used to indicate the optimal or natural pitch level, the fundamental frequencies were measured from spectrographs for this utterance prior to therapy and for numbers, reading, expressions, and vowels following therapy in 26 dysphonic patients (Cooper, 1972). In comparing the mean fundamental frequency of "um-hum" to the mean fundamental frequencies of reading, expression, vowels, and numbers in dysphonic groups of more than 2 patients, a difference of 0 to 1 semitone was noted in both male and female patients. In comparing the totals of the individual mean fundamental frequencies for reading, expression, numbers, and vowels after therapy for each patient to that patient's fundamental frequency for "um-hum" prior to therapy, a difference of 0 to 2 semitones was found in 21 of 26 patients. In this study, the clinical tool "um-hum" was found to afford a simple, direct method of locating natural or optimal pitch when utilized by a voice therapist knowledgeable in the use of this method.

The optimal pitch will assist the patient in achieving a proper tone focus, which is a balance of oronasopharyngeal resonance in combination with laryngeal resonance. There are kinesthetic and auditory cues to help recognize the proper tone focus which usually appears from use of the optimal pitch. Proper tone focus creates "sonorousness" (Tarneaud, 1958) or a "ring" (Cooper, 1971c). Zaliouk (1963, p. 149) notes that the optimal resonance pitch produces "optimal vibrations in the facial mask, which comprises the nose and maxillary bones." From clinical experience, the mask area also encompasses the lips as well as the sides and bridge of the nose. Tone focus in this area is called mask placement.

To help identify the placement of tone focus (and the optimal pitch), the fingers of one hand should be placed lightly on the bridge and sides of the nose while the other hand is placed lightly on the throat. As one says the "um-hum" there should be a slight vibration or tingle in the mask area. Some patients experience more vibration or tingle about the upper lip, while others experience the sensation around the bridge or sides of the nose. If there is too much laryngopharyngeal resonance, the pitch may be too low or the tone focus improperly placed in the throat.

This natural or "um-hum" method should not be confused with the experimental technique, described by Thurman (1958) and discussed by House (1959), which was to determine if the optimal pitch could be indicated by an involuntary swell of intensity. This author's natural or "um-hum" method elicits a spontaneous response and must depend to a degree on the trained ear of the therapist.

The ear of the voice therapist is, in the final analysis, the ultimate and decisive factor in the identification and maintenance of the optimal pitch level regardless of the exercise used to achieve the patient's producing the optimal pitch. The "um-hum" or natural method is also dependent upon the knowledgeable ear of the therapist, but this method can be used by less experienced therapists, if they are aware of the following conditions: (1) The "um-hum" must be spontaneous, sincere, and above all, natural. The therapist must recognize when it is natural. (2) The tone focus must be 50 percent in the mask area for oronasal resonance and 50 percent of the laryngopharynx area for lower throat resonance. If there is too much laryngopharyngeal resonance, then the pitch is probably too low; if there is a predominance of nasal resonance, the pitch may be too high.

Back-up methods to ascertain the optimal pitch level are as follows: (1) Ask the individual to say "hello" naturally (spontaneously and sincerely), with a rising inflection. Have him say this in a manner so as to reach the back of an audience. The "hello" with a rising inflection sounds like a question. (2) Have the patient say "me-me" or "nim-nim" naturally with both syllables on the same pitch level. (3) Listen to the natural, spontaneous laugh of the patient. The laugh, if not forced, is often representative of the optimal pitch level. It is easy to hear this spontaneous laughter during a conversation with the patient if one listens for it.

The key words, such as "um-hum," "me-me," and "nim-nim," utilized to find the optimal pitch level and proper tone focus are all nasal sounds or contain nasal consonants. This is done in order to place the tone focus in the oronasopharyngeal area, since most patients have too much laryngopharyngeal resonance and a basal or near basal pitch level. When the pitch range is too high, the "um-hum" once again affords a clear optimal pitch level. It has been found that the "um-hum" is spoken by most of these patients in their natural voice. Pahn (1964, p. 261-262) explains his rationale for the use of nasalized vowels:

> In the treatment of functional voice disorders exercises with na-salised vowels are shown to be helpful to most patients. . . . Apparently it is difficult or impossible for patients to nasalise vowels or vowel-like sounds and yet maintain the disturbed voice quality.

A technique which is helpful for a few patients who are too low in pitch is to go to the supraoptimal pitch level. The supraoptimal pitch level is one to three tones either at the highest tone in the optimal level (if the optimal pitch level is three tones) or at the tone directly above the optimal pitch level (if the optimal pitch level is one tone). The supraoptimal pitch level is used for some patients for the following reasons: (1) It takes the pressure off the laryngopharynx and very quickly alleviates or eliminates the vocal symptoms. This supraoptimal pitch produces a faster laryngeal and pharyngeal muscle re-alignment to normal muscular movement for voice. (2) Most patients have a tendency to drop in pitch from a given pitch level. If they are originally given a supraoptimal pitch level, when the pitch drop occurs, they will be at the optimal pitch level. If originally given the optimal pitch level, they tend to drop too far below the optimal pitch level. (3) The patient may not distinguish between the optimal pitch and the habitual pitch in the early stages of vocal rehabilitation. In the beginning of vocal therapy, the patient needs a wide difference between the two pitch levels. Therefore, if he is given a supraoptimal pitch level or higher pitch level initially, he can distinguish between the supraoptimal and the habitual pitch levels and hold to the supraoptimal pitch level easier.

The following types of patients are given a supraoptimal pitch level: (1) those who are unable to easily distinguish between the optimal pitch and the habitual pitch levels, (2) those who want immediate relief from vocal symptoms, and (3) those who want a rapid vocal rehabilitation process. Patients who utilize the supraoptimal pitch level must have the personality strength to hold to this pitch level in spite of any external reaction and internal concern. The internal reaction is more important than the external because the individual, in monitoring himself, may realize that there is a marked change in pitch and so tends to react to it. He believes that his internal reaction to the new pitch and new tone focus is similarly received by those about him. He soon realizes that others are essentially unaware of the new pitch and new tone focus which are fundamentally monitored by him alone. The immediate family, associates, or those with whom he communicates on the telephone may become aware of the new voice or new pitch, but they soon become accustomed to it and accepting of it.

While the new pitch and tone focus are being established, positive new vocal symptoms (alone or in combination) develop in addition to the initial or original negative vocal symptoms. The new pitch level and tone focus bring forth tension underneath the mandible, in the soft palate, and in the sternocleidomastoid muscle; a burning sensation in the soft palate; a sore throat; a tickling in the ear; and a movement of tension from the laryngopharynx to the oronasopharynx. These new symptoms disappear sometimes within a matter of days but more often within a matter of a few weeks to a few months, depending upon the consistency to which the patient utilizes the new pitch level.

The patient who reverts to the old habitual pitch may experience a combination of the original negative voice symptoms plus the new positive voice symptoms since he is utilizing both pitch levels. The return to the habitual pitch occurs either because the patient is unable to maintain the new pitch level or the patient becomes frightened and drops to the old pitch level when the new symptoms, caused by the new pitch level, appear. The patient must be forewarned that the new positive vocal symptoms will appear, that they are excellent signs of vocal improvement, and that they will be temporary. As the new voice is held, negative and positive pitch and focus symptoms should disappear. If any symptoms remain, the pitch or tone focus may still be incorrect. In a few patients, the continuance of negative vocal symptoms may be the result of psychological causes.

Voice breaks may occur during the development of the new pitch and tone focus. The patient must be reassured that pitch breaks are normal and short-lived.

Some patients feel that they are using a monotone voice while the optimal or supraoptimal pitch level is being mastered. These patients are assured that use of the limited pitch level is temporary and that vocal variety will soon be developed.

In the process of acquiring the new voice, the patient often finds his voice has a singsong quality. This is a normal and transitory stage. What sounds like singsong is more often than not a new exaggerated melodic and lilting inflection in the new voice created by use of the optimal pitch level or range.

Posturing may occur as the patient attempts to use the new pitch level and tone focus. Posturing is a form of imagery and may be internal or external. Imagery is a mental means a patient utilizes to define for himself the correct concept of pitch and tone focus. Patients vary in their ability to use imagery and in the type of imagery or mental picture which is utilized to help them achieve the proper pitch and tone focus. One patient visualizes talking through the top of his head; another sees the tone as being placed a short distance in front of the mouth; still another thinks of the sound as hitting the hard palate or upper teeth. The therapist affirms whether or not the imagery is producing the correct pitch and tone focus.

As the patient visualizes the pitch and tone focus in his mind's eye, he may use a physical internal or external posturing to achieve the proper sound. The internal posturing is important and of value to some patients. Internal posturing is the thought process used by the patient to help him better the pitch and the tone focus. Gross external posturing, or the way the patient keeps his head and shoulders, reinforces the new pitch and tone focus for some patients. Fine external posturing, such as the arching of the eyebrows or slight movement of the nose, is normal and helpful to some patients. Internal and external posturing are temporary. Van Riper and Irwin (1958) write that some patients need to use head tilting or laryngeal posture as a means of locating the desired pitch.

Exercises to Establish the Optimal Pitch and Tone Focus

The exercises given below are used to establish the optimal pitch level and the proper tone focus. A tape recorder or Language Master (Bell and Howell) is used for the recording and replay of these exercises.

Patients vary remarkably in their preference for a key word in the exercises. Most prefer "um-hum" or "me-me." One key word brings forth the optimal pitch level and tone focus better than another key word for different patients. The patient and the therapist decide which key word is best. This key word is used initially and as a reference point for all new exercises.

1. Key word and number exercises:
   (a) Say "um-hum one, um-hum two" to ten, with the number on the same pitch level as the "um-hum." Matching the pitch level of the number to the "um-hum" is more difficult than might be expected. The "um-hum" said with the mouth closed utilizes the natural tone focus; the number said with the mouth opened reverts to the old habitual pitch level, which the patient must avoid.
   (b) Say "nim-nim one, nim-nim two" to ten, again matching the "nim-nim" and the number in pitch and tone focus.
   (c) Use "me-me one, me-me two," to ten, as above.
2. After the key word and number exercises, the next step is to carry over the pitch level and tone focus into phrases or brief sentences.
   (a) Have the patient say, "me-me one, how are you?" "Me-me two, I am fine." "Me-me three, what time is it?" Me-me four, who said that?" The patient uses any phrases he wishes, as well as any key word, such as "me-me," or "nim-nim." Combining the key word and number exercises with the phrase gives the patient a reference point to transfer the pitch and tone focus to longer sentences.
   (b) The patient says the key word with the phrase, eliminating the number, such as "Me-me, I feel fine." "Me-

me, it is nice today." Again, any key word may be used, but the key word then remains the same throughout the exercise. Any phrase or brief sentence may be used.

(c) The patient continues the above exercise, switching to another key word. If he used "me-me," he may now change to "nim-nim" or "hello." The key words have different vowel sounds, and thus afford practice on various vowels and a carry-over of the pitch and tone focus from one vowel to another.

3. The patient next practices longer sentences from drill books, such as from Schoolfield (1951), Fairbanks (1960), or Eisenson (1965). He again says the key word prior to reading the sentence. He uses the same key word for a series of sentences and then changes to a new key word for the next group of sentences.

4. The patient talks spontaneously in sentences, saying a key word before or during or after each sentence.

5. The patient reads aloud from magazines with the pitch and tone focus being monitored by the patient and the therapist.

6. The patient talks spontaneously to the therapist, who routinely reminds the patient if the pitch and tone focus are incorrect. Those few patients who have been utilizing the supraoptimal pitch level are now lowered in pitch to the optimal pitch level. Steps 5 and 6 may occur concomitantly.

7. The patient has been attempting since the beginning of therapy to use the new pitch level in the therapy session and outside the therapy session. The patient is usually much more successful in using the pitch level in the office than outside the office. The final step is a carry-over of the correct pitch level and tone focus to all situations.

The key words, especially "um-hum," may be used in all situations as a reminder of the proper pitch level and tone focus. This word is said spontaneously as if the patient were acknowledging a comment or agreeing with what was said. Since the "um-hum" is socially acceptable, it can be used unobtrusively in conversation as a therapeutic maneuver such as in the following example: "I understand (um-hum) that you might consider tak-

ing the time (um-hum) to go home next year for a vacation."
The patient may use this device at any time when he feels he
has lost the proper pitch level or tone focus.

If the patient has a morning voice upon arising, he should
raise the pitch immediately by the use of the "um-hum" or another exercise. The patient should not continue to utilize the
low pitch of the morning voice.

Patients progress at different rates in the process of establishing the optimal pitch and tone focus. Some are able to quickly
master the mechanical exercises in the beginning of therapy, but
have more difficulty with carry-over in the later stages. Other patients must practice the mechanical exercises for a long period
of time, but the carry-over is relatively easy and accomplished
in a short period of time.

Exercises for Tone Focus

In most patients, the pitch and tone focus are interdependent.
In the misused voice, the pitch is usually within the basal range
and the tone focus is within the laryngopharynx. When the
pitch level is raised to the optimal pitch level, the tone focus is
usually changed to a balanced oronasopharyngeal resonance.
However, in some patients the pitch and tone focus operate in-
dependently. The pitch may be raised to the optimal pitch level,
but the tone focus remains within the laryngopharynx. The optimal pitch affords some oronasal resonance but not enough.
These patients are extremely difficult to work with. Their basic
problem is one of resonance balance. Nasal resonance is stressed
at first, followed by an adjustment of the tone focus to a balanced oronasopharyngeal resonance.

These patients have a strong negative vocal image regarding
nasal resonance. They feel that nasal resonance means nasality
and that they are developing a nasal voice by placing the resonance in an area other than the laryngopharynx. They must be
reassured the voice is not nasal.

Exercises to place the tone focus in the nasopharynx are as
follows:

1. Use the vowel /i/ or (ē) in combination with consonants or
alone, such as "e-e," "me-me," "ne-ne," "he-he."

2. Combine the vowel or the syllable with a number, such as "e one, e two," "me one, me two."

3. Combine the vowel or syllable with a word, next with a phrase, followed by the use of sentences and paragraphs.

4. Incorporate the correct tone focus in spontaneous speech.

Severe Dysphonia

In a limited number of patients, the vocal fold(s) is impaired to the degree that the patient is severely dysphonic. Although the patient is able to phonate, he may be unable to phonate a sufficient number of pitches for the therapist to be able to locate the optimal pitch. If so, the patient is directed to practice the exercises described below gently until the voice returns. This may be a period of several weeks or longer if the pathology is extremely severe. This protracted period of time to regain a pitch range is infrequent and occurs in most cases only following a surgical procedure, such as bilateral stripping of the vocal folds in polypoid degeneration.

The patient practices these exercises at home five to fifteen minutes on the hour, as many times per day as is possible. The patient should be forewarned that the sound may come in slowly or that the voice may develop over a period of time. The patient should not be discouraged if he remains nearly aphonic for a period of two to four weeks in some cases. He should continue practicing the exercises as described below.

1. The patient prolongs the vowel /o/ starting at the top of his pitch range and extending to the bottom of the pitch range, attempting to slide through as many notes as possible throughout the range. The patient must phonate gently and not force the voice or use volume.

2. The patient repeats the above exercise, starting at the bottom of the pitch range and progressing to the top, remembering to prolong the vowel in a slur effect.

3. The patient repeats the two exercises above using the vowels, /i/, /u/, /a/. One vowel may be more productive of sound than another; this vowel should be utilized more than the other vowels. The vowel /a/ is the most difficult to produce on a sliding scale for dysphonic patients.

4. As soon as the patient is able to phonate an extended series of pitches, the therapist attempts to locate the optimal pitch level in the usual manner previously described.

5. The patient uses a vowel, such as /o/, and starting at the top of his pitch range, produces the vowel four or five times at this level and on each successive pitch level down to the bottom of his pitch range.

6. The patient repeats the above exercise, starting at the bottom of his pitch range and repeating a vowel several times on each pitch level as he progresses to the top of his pitch range.

7. The patient practices the above exercises, using different vowels, such as /i/, /a/, and /u/.

8. The patient repeats the above exercises, using a different vowel on each step or pitch level. Depending upon the individual patient, the sequence of exercises 6 through 9 may be practiced following exercises 10 through 13. Exercises 9 through 13 are optional.

9. The patient changes vowels as he prolongs the sound from the top to the bottom of his pitch range and then from the bottom to the top, such as /o/, /i/, /a/, or other combinations. The patient should use vowel combinations which allow him to achieve sound in vowels which he has not been able to produce with sound previously. An example would be /i/ sound easily produced; /a/ difficult to achieve sound; /o/ sound easily produced.

10. The patient phonates the vowel /o/ from the top of the pitch range to the bottom, producing the vowel step-by-step on each pitch level down the scale, instead of slurring or prolonging the vowel as was done previously.

11. The patient repeats the above exercise, going from the bottom to the top of the pitch range.

12. The patient repeats the two exercises above using different vowels, such as /u/, /i/, /a/.

13. The patient changes vowels as he progresses from the top to the bottom and bottom to the top of the pitch range, using a different vowel on each step or pitch level.

The therapist may find that the patient can produce a combination of one or two consonants with a vowel easier than a vowel in isolation. If so, the patient is directed to practice the exercises using syllables such as "me," "no," "ne," "zim," "nim," and "nem." The patient may prefer to use the sound "um-hum." Examples of these exercises are given below.

14. The patient produces a continuous sound of "me" on a sliding scale from the top to the bottom of the pitch range and from the bottom to the top.

15. The patient gently produces "me-me one" to ten on each pitch level starting at the highest comfortable pitch level and moving down the pitch range one step at a time to the lowest comfortable pitch level.

16. The patient practices the above exercise starting at the lowest pitch level and moving gently without forcing to the highest pitch level.

17. The patient repeats the above exercises with a change in the vowel or consonant, such as "mo-mo one," "moo-moo one," "ma-ma one," "ne-ne one," or "nim-nim one."

Pitch Discrimination

Some authors report that voice problems are the result of poor pitch discrimination. Eisenson, Kastein, and Schneiderman (1958, p. 581) state:

> According to the results of this study, voice defectives appear to be inferior in pitch discrimination as compared to the normal population. It may be theorized that poor pitch discrimination can be a causal factor in the development of voice disorders associated with poor pitch placement. . . .

These authors did note that 15 patients receiving therapy showed significant gain in pitch discrimination. Fisher (in Gildston and Gildston 1968, p. 125) states: "Our research with auditory perception tends to indicate that patients with habitual hyperkinetic dysphonia have poorest pitch perception and therefore are possibly lest [sic] trainable in changing pitch for speech." However, Davis and Boone (1967) indicate that patients with hyperfunctional voice problems, such as vocal nodules, cord thickening, contact ulcers, and dysphonia without laryngeal pathology, are similar to the normal population in pitch discrimination and memory of tonal sequence. Riker (1946) writes that the ability to judge pitch is not confined to specially trained or musically talented individuals. Heinberg (1964, p. 188) states: "Ninety-five percent of a group can produce a wide variety of pitches accurately."[*]

Clinical experience indicates that initially voice patients vary markedly in their ability to perceive different pitch levels. The vast majority are quickly able to discriminate correct from incorrect pitch levels and ranges. Only a handful of patients seen might be categorized as tone-deaf. Even these managed to master an efficient voice in due time. In clinical voice therapy, the concern is with the patient's ability to monitor his optimal pitch in continuous speech, not with determining pitch differences between two or more pure tones in laboratory tests. Ear training by tape replay and by repeated specific direction by the therapist guides the patient to perceive differences in pitch levels and to monitor his own given optimal pitch. The view that voice patients are defective in pitch discrimination is a myth if clinical experience is to be considered.

Quality

The new pitch and tone focus develop a new quality of voice. This new voice quality may initially emphasize nasal resonance. The new voice quality is not nasal, but when there has previously been a dearth or absence of nasal resonance, the patient may perceive the new nasal resonance as nasality. The patient must be shown that nasal resonance is not nasality. Weiss, a discussant in Vennard (1962, p. 419) quotes Reszke, who remarked: "The sound should be in the nose but the nose should not be in the sound." The use of the Language Master for constant replay of the voice, using the new pitch and tone focus, soon accustoms the patient to the new sound. The new voice is also discussed from the point of view of the new vocal image and the new vocal identity.

In the very early stages of tone focus therapy, the patient may have the tendency once he accedes to or accepts the concept of nasal resonance to overstress nasal resonance so that nasality is produced. This nasality is quickly dissipated. The patient is cautioned not to react negatively to comments of outsiders at this

---

[*] Paul Heinberg, *Voice Training,* Copyright 1964, Ronald Press Co., New York.

stage. This transition from incorrect to correct tone focus may create excessive nasopharyngeal resonance in some patients.

The new pitch level and tone focus will eliminate most deviant voice qualities. If the quality is nasal, lowering the pitch level, in most cases, will eliminate the nasality, as a lower pitch affords more oral and laryngeal resonance. If the quality is hoarse, harsh, or breathy, a raised pitch level and a tone focus in the mask area will usually resolve the problem of quality.

In a study by this author (1972) hoarseness was objectively determined from spectrographic analysis of 3 vowels before therapy by using the categories established by Yanagihara (1962) to classify hoarseness into four types, Type I (slight) through Type IV (severe). After therapy the vowels were analyzed by using two additional types established for this study, Type 0+ to indicate a trace of hoarseness (less than Type I) and Type 0 to indicate no hoarseness (clear voice). Prior to therapy, all patients exhibited hoarseness in the vowels in varying degrees. Following therapy, hoarseness was basically eliminated in all patients, with the exception of a trace of hoarseness or slight hoarseness in one vowel in a few patients. One other aspect should be noted. In studying the relationship prior to therapy between fundamental frequencies and hoarseness in dysphonic males and females, the patients who had the lowest fundamental frequencies for vowels exhibited hoarseness of Types III and IV, while patients with the highest fundamental frequencies for vowels had hoarseness of Types I and II.

Volume

Most voice patients lack volume or the ability to produce volume easily, without strain and without discomfort. Few voice cases present a problem of too much volume. The lack of volume is usually due to an incorrect tone focus and pitch level. Laryngopharyngeal resonance and basal pitch do not carry.

When the voice patient begins therapy, he usually has too little volume. The patient may need more volume in order to produce the optimal pitch level and the proper tone focus. As soon as the correct tone focus and pitch level are located and established, the patient may feel that he has too much volume. Oronasopharyngeal resonance when correctly balanced affords a great deal of carrying power to the voice. Because of the additional volume used to produce the optimal pitch and because of the carrying power of the new pitch and balanced tone focus, the patient may feel that he is shouting as he produces the new voice. The patient reacts critically to the new and additional volume. Actually, most patients are not loud at all, but when patients compare the old voice which had no carrying power to the new voice which does have carrying power, they are loud. In essence, they are really normal in volume with the new voice. They hear themselves as loud through the bones of their head and fail to realize that listeners do not hear them as loud; it is their own monitoring system which makes them sound loud to themselves. Reassurance from the therapist, acceptance from friends and associates, and repeated tape replays are means of affording the patient insight and understanding that his new volume is normal and that he is not shouting.

Some patients develop too much volume as they develop a new voice. In the early stages of rehabilitation, volume is an essential adjunct to developing and maintaining the new tone focus and pitch level. Once they have achieved the new pitch and level and tone focus, volume may need to be reduced. Since most conversation does not require much volume, it is necessary to direct the patient to a moderate volume in voice. Patients must be taught to contain additional volume, or else they are wasting their effort and their volume pointlessly.

Some patients have no difficulty using the new voice in normal circumstances. When they try to increase the volume in a noisy atmosphere or to be heard at a distance, they may pitch the voice too high or too low and use the lower laryngopharyngeal area for tone focus. These individuals need to learn how to project the speaking voice by emphasizing oronasopharyngeal resonance and using an optimal pitch with midsection breath support.

Other patients require a great deal of volume in voice. They, of necessity, have to compete with noise during work or recreational activities. In order to produce loud but natural volume, midsection breath support and projection also must be taught the patient. (See Special Needs—projection.)

Those individuals who have too much volume must learn to reduce the volume and must understand why they are loud and what need the loud voice fulfills within them. The vast majority of individuals with volume problems, whether they are too loud or too soft, lack a correct tone focus and pitch level. They therefore experience vocal strain and many other vocal symptoms of a voice disorder. Some of the individuals do have a well-focused and well-pitched voice and merely require vocal psychotherapy which helps them to use adequate volume.

Breath Support

Nearly all voice patients lack proper midsection breath support for speech. Midsection breath support for speech allows for properly controlled air usage. It also takes the muscular tension away from the laryngeal and pharyngeal area, placing it on the abdominal muscles, which are much more able to bear pressure and tension without interfering with vocalization. One should bear in mind that the laryngeal and pharyngeal tensions experienced by voice patients disappear when midsection breath support is mastered along with the correct tone focus and pitch level. Midsection breath support also allows for controlled volume without undue effort. Those who have upper chest or clavicular breathing for speech squeeze out the tone or voice when they are involved in producing an effortful voice.

Very often breath support is the final step in the resolution of a voice disorder. It must not be developed in the early stages of vocal rehabilitation, or else the patient will have too much volume with an incorrect tone focus and pitch level, which will further aggravate the voice. The essential elements in overcoming most negative vocal symptoms revolve about the proper tone focus and pitch level. The remaining negative vocal symptoms, lack of carrying power and laryngeal and pharyngeal neck tensions, can be eliminated by the mastering of midsection breath support. Midsection breath support is necessary for adults and children who require easy, comfortable volume for specific or general circumstances. Unfortunately, not all children have the patience or the time, nor do all therapists have the ability to teach the child how to develop midsection breath support.

Clinical experience indicates that voice patients learn midsection breath support best in a given programmed sequential order:

1. The patient lies in a supine position, with one hand on his chest and the other on his stomach. The patient gently breathes in through his nostrils. There is no need or point to breathing in deeply. The patient breathes in only as he has need for air for vegetative or survival purposes. The midsection or stomach moves outward with the chest remaining stationary during inhalation. The patient exhales through his mouth. During exhalation, the midsection smoothly and slowly deflates. The patient next inhales through the mouth (instead of through the nose) and exhales again through the mouth. Breathing is gentle, not labored nor forced.

2. The patient repeats the above sequence in a standing position, again keeping one hand on the chest and the other on the stomach. The procedure is inhaling through the nose and exhaling through the mouth, followed by inhaling and exhaling both through the mouth. During this portion of the exercise, the midsection should expand and deflate gently and smoothly.

3. The patient again repeats the sequence, this time in a sitting position, which is the most difficult position in the mastery of midsection breath support.

4. The patient is placed in a sitting position at the Language Master or tape recorder. He inhales through his nose and counts aloud "me-me one, me-me two, me-me three" and exhales through his mouth. Thus, he is able to feel the midsection expand on inhalation and deflate on exhalation. The patient repeats the above, this time inhaling through the mouth. The inhalation must be moderate and natural, or else the mucous lining of the throat will be dried by a deep breath. A deep breath will also tense the entire body for those who are learning midsection breath support.

5. Through recording and replay, the patient learns to keep the proper pitch level, tone focus, quality, and volume by using "me-me one, me-me two," or "nim-nim one, nim-nim two." The patient usually loses the correct production of these elements as he works on midsection breath support. The patient is advised this is temporary and basically inevitable.

6. When the midsection breath support is mastered in mechanical exercises, the patient begins to work at breath support in spontaneous phrases and sentences. The patient can monitor his midsection support by keeping one hand on his midsection as he inhales and exhales throughout the training procedure.

7. The final stage of midsection breath support is also the final stage for pitch level, tone focus, quality, and volume. These elements are coordinated as the patient and therapist converse in spontaneous speech with both the patient and the therapist monitoring the patient's breath support as well as the other vocal elements of voice.

Some patients prefer to avoid the automation approach, that is the use of the Language Master or tape recorder, and simply converse with the therapist for those stages originally using the Language Master.

Hyperventilation or excessive oxygen intake is experienced during the early stages of mechanical breathing exercises and some patients may become dizzy. The patient should be cautioned to attend to the exercises easily and regularly. Many patients have the tendency to run through the exercises too quickly in anticipation that such activity will speed up the therapy and afford them faster results.

Rate

Some patients find it is easier to slow the rate as they master the various elements of voice. Others find it more expedient to speed up the rate of speech as they work on the various elements of voice. Rate of speech is an individual matter and the patient should be allowed to utilize whatever rate is comfortable and natural during the vocal rehabilitative process. For the most part, patients usually slow down the rate, as they are unable to concentrate on the process and the content at the same time. For those who practice at a slower rate, the normal rate is resumed once the various elements of voice are combined and coordinated properly. A patient who had a fast rate prior to therapy may find that the concentration upon the process of vocal rehabilitation will slow the rate, so that following the completion of vocal rehabilitation the rate remains permanently slower.

If the patient has a problem of rate, the rate must be worked on from a mechanistic point of view and without concentration on other elements of voice. The satisfactions achieved from a fast or slow rate must be analyzed fully, as rate may reflect a personality need and fulfillment. Rate may also be a habit, learned from imitation or from necessity. The therapeutic approach to the problem of rate depends upon the analysis of factors causing the deviant rate.

Carry-over of the New Voice

In carry-over of the new voice from the office or therapy situation to outside situations, the patient progresses in steps. At first, the patient learns only pitch and tone focus and works on carry-over of these variables. As he learns to control volume and breath support, he must also practice carry-over of these elements.

The carry-over from the therapy sessions to outside situations will be gradual, not spontaneous. The responsibility for holding the new voice throughout the day is basically dependent upon the patient's own ego strength. Individuals will vary in their abilities to transfer the new voice to outside situations.

Peripatetic vocal carry-over is used with patients who are more comfortable outside of the office and who enjoy walking. Some patients prefer visits to restaurants for coffee during therapy. These therapy situations are used in combination with office therapy. At all times, the therapist is monitoring the patient's voice in spontaneous conversation and is making suggestions for vocal improvement.

In the carry-over of the new voice from office therapy to outside situations, many patients find that they cannot easily concentrate upon using the new voice without interfering with what they have to say. The *how* or the manner of using the voice is interfering with the *what* or the content of speech. Usually the transition is gradual and in the main, progressive, but there are lapses and failures toward the maintenance of the new voice in variable situations.

Some patients can use the new voice when they are alone or not under pressure. When they are with others or feel pressure they have little confidence in their new voice and are unable to use it constantly.

The patient must learn to overcome vocal self-consciousness about the new voice. The new voice must be used outside the therapy session and accepted as a new and real voice. It must not be considered a phony or put-on voice.

Vocal concentration upon the new voice is fatiguing if not exhausting. Depending upon the patient's state of health, age, and the kind of therapy (regular or intensive) the fatigue or exhaustion will be accentuated accordingly during the process of vocal rehabilitation. Overcoming a voice problem is hard work, requiring physical, mental, and emotional effort.

One patient explained:

> You have to talk yourself into it. You work at it, and keep at it, and try hard until it becomes natural and second nature. Then, when you have accomplished it, you are fine. But no one really knows how hard you worked at it because they don't see it in writing. They only hear a new voice.

Only a few people associated with the patient who know that he is undergoing vocal therapy realize that his voice is different. Most individuals around the patient are unaware of the change in voice. While many individuals notice adverse or negative effects upon the voice, such as hoarseness, a cold, or fatigue, most people do not seem to notice an improvement in voice.

Tape Replay

Tape replay of the patient's old voice and new voice as he progresses in therapy is vital. Frequent practice with a recording device is also necessary.

Weston and Rousey (1970) theorize that the use of the tape recorder in clinical practice is tenuous at best. They (p. 552) write: ". . . there is little evidence to support the assumption that confronting oneself with an undesirable behavior and possibly comparing it to a desirable one should lead a reasonable person to prompt modification of his undesirable behavior." However, most authors do not agree with this view. In fact, the great majority recommend and use tape recordings.

Van Riper and Irwin (1958) advise frequent playbacks of the old and new voices since the new pitch often causes the patient to feel strange and uncomfortable. Williamson (1945, p. 196) finds:

Nothing proved more useful than the motivation that resulted from the student's being able to compare his voice, after he had made some improvement, with his original recording. This was the proof of the pudding, which generally changed an initial attitude of unconvinced reluctance to that of cooperation or even enthusiasm.

Knower and Emerson (1946) indicate the need for before and after tapes to determine progress and that the recordings show achievement. Henrikson and Irwin (1949, p. 232) state: "Voice recording is here as a legitimate and valuable part of speech correction. The question is not one of blind acceptance but of analysis for maximum use."

The approach to vocal rehabilitation that affords the patient no opportunity to compare the initial recordings of the voice and periodic reevaluations of the voice as therapy proceeds is without any point and any premise other than opinion. Only when the therapist is unsure of his ability to improve the voice is it perhaps best that comparative tapes not be afforded the patient.

The use of the tape machine is undesirable if it is not properly used. Having a patient listen to his misused and poor voice without basic and concrete hope for improvement can be devastating.

Unguided therapy or self-direction when using the tape machine can be extremely dangerous. Some patients have altered the basic pitch and tone focus of the speaking voice because of the tape replay. These patients hear their voices as thin, lacking in richness, or too high. They pitch the voice lower and seek a fuller sound with laryngopharyngeal resonance. Tape replay and do-it-yourself therapy without competently guided voice direction can create voice disorders.

Tape replay has been an integral part of this author's vocal rehabilitation program and has been extremely successful in making the patient recognize and accept the need for vocal rehabilitation. Those who maintain that tape replay is embarrassing or terrifying to the patient may cite selected instances. Given the chance to hear himself the voice patient almost inevitably approves of this approach. Of approximately 1400 consecutive patients with voice disorders seen covering a period of ten years, not more than a miniscule number declined to listen to the replay and subsequent replays estimating the vocal progress. These 1400 voice cases support the view that not only has tape replay had no harmful effects upon patients, but also that tape replay is a necessary requirement in therapy for helping patients gain better vocal awareness and vocal improvement.

Awareness of the voice problem, which is underscored for the patient by a tape replay, is essential if anything at all is to be done for the patient. In most cases, when the patient begins voice therapy, he is unaware of how he actually sounds unless he has previously heard himself on a tape recorder. When he hears his own voice played back, he is usually surprised and often fails to recognize it as his voice. He dislikes the voice he hears; he is disdainful of it. In a limited survey of 70 patients selected at random from patient files, only 10 out of 70 recognized their voices when the tape was replayed. Voice awareness and vocal consciousness must be taught. It takes time and effort for a therapist to train a patient to hear himself. It is important to use a tape machine of good fidelity so that the patient can hear himself correctly and learn to recognize his own voice.

There is need for playback before, during, and after therapy. Some patients require numerous replays comparing the original voice to the new voice during therapy. Many suffice with a few replays. The frequency of the replays and comparisons is dependent upon the needs of the individual patient. Comments by patients reinforce the necessity for tape replays. One patient said: "When I talk at this new pitch level, it sounds strained to me. But you know something? When I hear it back, it sounds okay."

In this author's therapy approach, the patient's habitual voice is recorded during the initial interview on a master tape and on one track of several Language Master cards. As vocal progress is made, the new voice is superimposed upon the original recording and on the second track of the cards for easy comparison. The new voice compared to the old (original) voice is evidence of the extent of vocal improvement and is the convincing aspect of vocal therapy. The new voice further encourages the patient to work harder toward a complete resolution. The comparative recording also establishes within the patient's mind the inefficient sound that was his original voice. From the original tape and the new superimposed voice, the patient hears himself as he was and as he is. If the therapist has done a creditable job, the difference is marked and the patient is aware of his vocal improvement.

Without a comparison of the old and new voices, the patient may denigrate his vocal progress. Many patients forget how poor their old voices were and how bad they sounded. Upon hearing the old voice after the new voice is established, patients often comment, "Did I sound that bad?" They are unable to remember. That is why it is imperative to always replay the original voice and compare it to the new voice via superimpositions upon the original tape. Our clinical research and experience in using the tape recorder and other recording devices with voice patients completely affirms the appropriateness and need for the use of recording to alter vocal patterns.

Automation Carry-over Techniques

An essential device for pitch, tone focus, and quality feedback to the patient is the Bell and Howell Language Master. The Language Master has a two track recording system that uses a card with a recording tape on it. The quality reproduction of the Language Master is excellent.

In the initial session on one track of several Language Master cards, the patient records spontaneous speech at his habitual pitch level. During this session and during later therapy sessions on the other track of several cards, the patient records "nim-nim one," "me-me one," or "um-hum one" to ten. He listens to these latter tracks with the therapist. They agree or disagree upon the patient's ability to produce the correct pitch level, tone focus, and quality and to transfer these elements from the key word to the number. The patient remains at this exercise until he masters the production of the new pitch, tone focus, and quality. Volume may also be monitored by keeping the volume control of the Language Master constant and by having the patient remain an indicated distance from the machine.

Periodically, depending upon individual needs, the patient listens to the difference between the old habitual voice and the new voice by changing tracks as the cards move through the Language Master. The patient must hear the two voices in order to identify the correct and incorrect vocal production. No amount of verbalization alone about the new voice as compared to the old voice suffices.

Some patients rent or buy the machine in order to practice at home to afford a better and quicker carry-over from the therapy session to the home. The long cards must be utilized; the short cards do not afford enough time for the patient to record and to hear the two voices by changing tracks as the card moves through the machine.

Automation in the form of the Language Master or tape recorder may be used appropriately. Some patients are highly negative to the use of any continued mechanical device. The therapist must work directly with these patients, being a monitor and guiding them to the correct pitch and tone focus. This process usually takes longer.

Most patients can benefit from the use of automation. They learn to identify, isolate, and establish the proper pitch level, tone focus, quality, and volume, later combining these elements with midsection breath support through the use of the Language Master, and thereby speed up the rehabilitative process.

VOCAL PSYCHOTHERAPY

Psychotherapy may be defined as an attempt to undo, modify, or resolve a disorder or problem which is adversely affecting an individual. Interpersonal therapy which is being afforded by a mature and competent therapist is essentially psychotherapy. Vocal psychotherapy is psychotherapy which revolves around the vocal aspects of the individual, his personality, his background, his environment, and his culture.

Personality needs may play a part in the establishment or continuation of a voice disorder. This factor may be major or minor in the constellation of the onset and development of dysphonias and of their treatment. The voice therapist must be able to refashion the patient's voice, his concepts of it, and his use of it, so that a clear easy voice is produced and habituated. As Anderson (1961, p. 9) states: "Thus, in a sense, voice training is personality training, in the same way that personality training is also voice training." Vocal rehabilitation provides the opportunity for an individual to develop his personality and fulfill his vocal potential.

Voice patients generally fall into four categories: (1) Those with a voice disorder and little or no psychological involvement. These patients can be treated by vocal rehabilitation and vocal psychotherapy. (2) Those with a voice disorder and an accompanying unrelated psychological involvement which is not being affected by the voice disorder and not affecting the voice disorder. These patients can overcome their voice disorder through vocal rehabilitation and vocal psychotherapy. The psychological problem may remain, but it may be modified or eliminated through insights gained in vocal psychotherapy. (3) Those with a voice disorder and a psychological problem which is being created and continued by the voice disorder. These patients are given vocal rehabilitation and vocal psychotherapy. The elimination of the voice disorder removes the activating cause of the psychological problem. Vocal psychotherapy usually completes the rehabilitative process. (4) Those patients with a voice disorder and a psychological problem which is creating and continuing the voice disorder. These patients are few in number, but most of them need psychotherapy to resolve their psychological problems prior to or concomitant with vocal rehabilitation. At some point vocal rehabilitation with vocal psychotherapy is necessary, since psychotherapy alone will not remove the voice disorder.

Relevance and Techniques of Vocal Psychotherapy

Vocal psychotherapy, brief or extended, is imperative and inherent within the process of vocal rehabilitation once the vocal image has been created and established because (1) the vocal image is often contributory to the onset and development of the voice disorder; (2) the vocal image is the most vital and pervasive psychological factor in the resolution and termination of the voice disorder; and (3) the vocal image is seriously resistant to change, regardless of the patient's intellectual understanding of its initial formation and development in regard to his voice. The ability of the therapist to impress these facts upon the patient and the patient's intellectual and emotional realization and acceptance of change regarding the vocal image are among the keys to the reversal of the voice disorder.

Almost all voice patients have one form or another of the vocal image. Individuals may consciously espouse a given voice for purposes of fulfilling themselves, and when such is the case, this consideration must be understood. When the vocal image is created out of ignorance and misconception of the proper use of the voice, the individual may be more amenable to direct vocal rehabilitation and the extent of therapy is usually reduced.

It is not possible to determine initially just which vocal image and which voice patient involved will yield to vocal psychotherapy. Three factors must be determined and considered regardless of the originating cause of the vocal image: (1) the extent of the image or the length of time that the vocal image has prevailed; (2) its positive and negative attributes as measured in terms of the patient and his circumstances; and (3) the support and the need fulfillment it has provided its user.

It may be difficult to alter a vocal image—a voice of authority or a confidential voice—when that voice has provided satisfactions and positive aspects to the speaker for a long period of time or when such satisfactions are intense and rewarding. The vocal image must be productive of enough extended negative symptoms to encourage and incite the voice patient to seek and to continue voice therapy. A vocal image created only a year ago may well be resistant to vocal therapy, including vocal psychotherapy, because of its measurable positive factors to the patient and the absence or limited number of negative vocal symptoms. The incorrect use of pitch or tone focus for one year does not allow sufficient time for the negative vocal symptoms to occur and to be an influence for that individual to change his voice and his vocal image. The voice disorder must be chronic or periodically acute for the most part to activate the voice patient to consider vocal therapy in the first place.

Discussion and analysis of the old vocal image, which may have contributed to the onset of the voice disorder, is usually begun in the first session. By old vocal image is meant the image which has resulted in shaping the patient's current voice.

In the subsequent sessions, the discussion of the old vocal image and old voice continues. The patient's awareness must be brought to the factors which shaped the old vocal image and the old voice. The relationship of the patient's voice to the voices of family members, if and when such relationships exist, must be clearly detailed for the patient. The influence of society, via the mass media and the vocal neurosis which stress the low-pitched voice as a premium type of communication, must be afforded the patient. The need of the patient to acquiesce to social pressures and seek counterfeit maturity, sophistication, authority, relaxation and covert or overt sexuality through the voice must be made clear to the patient. The patient's correlation of a low-pitched voice with the representation of external security to buttress internal insecurity must be resolved.

The vocal image, then, is a key factor in all individuals undergoing vocal rehabilitation, since patients decline to change a voice when it does not meet with their aesthetic or preconceived sound concept. The vocal image may be so strongly rooted in the individual that any attempt to alter the image by altering the pitch, tone focus, or volume creates immediate and exaggerated concern by the individual toward the new voice. Weiss (1955, p. 213) states: "Although we may assume that it constitutes a general rule that the individual does not know his own voice, he must have a very concrete relation to it because patients violently resist any change of their vocal functioning brought about by therapeutic intervention."

Patients, male or female, adult or adolescent, react most strongly to an alteration in pitch and tone focus, regardless of how limited that change may be. Pitch change to the optimal pitch level initiates an immediate response, nearly always negative. For a male who has too low a pitch, the new higher pitch creates a feeling and an emotional response that this new pitch sounds squeaky, phoney, affected, or effeminate. Females react to the higher pitch as sounding shrewish, childish, or sharp. For men who have a falsetto voice, the lower optimal pitch sounds hoarse, unnatural, or strained. The younger patient does not react negatively quite as openly toward the new pitch as does the adult.

Factors influencing the rejection of a new pitch are (1) difficulty in identifying and maintaining it during and after the therapy session; (2) lack of familiarity with the correct pitch mechanistically and pragmatically which make it too troublesome and experimental for the patient to quickly use, accept, and control; (3) lack of control of the new pitch; and (4) fear of critical reactions to the new pitch.

A psychological consideration is that the individual identifies with his pitch. A change in pitch may denote a change of personality to the patient. Therefore, he attempts to maintain the established pitch, though that pitch level and range are revealed to him as inappropriate and productive of his voice disorder.

The patient's reaction to the new pitch is mollified by tape replay of the new voice and the new pitch. At first, the patient often states that he hears himself as sounding higher pitched than he really is with the new pitch level. Air conduction playback via the Language Master and tape recorder alerts the patient to the fact that the pitch is not as high as he initially believed it was. The patient's hypercritical reaction of the elevation of pitch or the lowering of the pitch for falsetto patients is further decreased by minimal or absence of outside reaction from intimate family members, friends, associates, and acquaintances.

If the voice patient insists upon maintaining the misused and inappropriate pitch level as sacrosanct, regardless of therapeutic endeavors, therapy must emphasize vocal psychotherapy. The patient's inability or disability to confront his voice problem realistically and meet the physical change of voice necessary to improve underscores the extent and involvement of the pitch factor with the personality needs and demands. It may also define the patient's lack of insight and relevance that pitch plays in the onset and development of a voice disorder. A change in pitch level and range is not immediately accepted or utilized by most voice patients. They must be conditioned and repeatedly encouraged by the therapist to seek, use, and enjoy the new pitch.

Nearly all voice patients resist the change in tone focus from excessive laryngopharyngeal resonance to balanced oronasopharyngeal resonance. The fear of sounding nasal prevails in almost all patients. The voice patient learning to place the tone focus in the mask feels and hears it as being nasal. He misinterprets nasal resonance as nasality. The connotation and the denotation of nasality is so repulsive and so great a deterrent to voice patients that this aspect of the vocal image must be clearly defined to the patient. He must understand that he will not sound nasal during and following the completion of the vocal rehabilitation process.

As the new voice and new vocal image begin to develop, discussion of the following aspects is necessary. The new voice and new vocal image are productive of external and internal stresses. The patient fears the new voice given to him by the voice therapist as being radically different from the old voice, be it pitch, tone focus, quality, or any other aspect. He not only fears the reaction of others toward the new sound or voice but also fears his own internal reaction toward the new voice. He hears the new voice or tone through the bones of his head and is unable to grasp and reconcile the fact that the way he hears his new voice and the way listeners hear the new voice are essentially two different matters. The patient feels that his old voice has positive qualities and that the new voice may not have these qualities. He fears the new voice does not represent his personality and his body image. He also fears losing control of his voice and is concerned that his new voice might break or lack the control of the old voice. The patient does not fully understand or accept the fact that the new voice and new vocal image will alleviate or eliminate the voice problem. He, therefore, emotionally resists changing his voice until he finds reassurance from others as well as from the therapist that the new voice is right for him. The patient must always understand through vocal psychotherapy that the new voice *is* right for him.

As the patient begins to accept the new voice and the new vocal image and to reject the old voice and the old vocal image, he experiences a vocal identity crisis, which may be brief or extended. The voice therapist must provide careful guidance through the vocal identity crisis as well as understanding of the personality effect of the new voice and new vocal identity to prevent the voice patient from lapsing back into the old voice. The therapist must understand the extremely strong influences that the vocal image and the vocal role play upon and within the voice patient. The alteration in vocal image requires time, patience, insight, and understanding by both the voice therapist and the patient.

Vocal Self-consciousness in Vocal Rehabilitation

Patients in vocal rehabilitation are extremely self-conscious about how they sound to others and to themselves when they are practicing a new sound. The therapist must make the patient feel at ease while performing the exercises necessary for location and establishment of the proper pitch and tone focus and while practicing the new voice. Assurance that all patients have to undergo a similar process of training allows the patient to feel part of a larger group. He can identify with them and avoid considering himself as unique in his needs and vocal behavior.

Vocal self-consciousness is an important transitory stage experienced by all patients. It is an essential aspect of vocal progress and varies in extent and duration among voice patients. Therapy is incomplete until the patient passes through this stage and eliminates all vocal self-consciousness about his new voice.

Vocal Catharsis

Vocal catharsis is part of voice therapy. Patients need vocal catharsis. During the therapy sessions, the patient must have the opportunity to express his vocal views, to have these concepts approved or denied and, thereby, to form a vocal philosophy that is substantial and meaningful to him for life situations. Until and unless such vocal catharsis is experienced, vocal training will remain superficial and pointless to the demanding voice patient.

Vocal Cues

Voice patients may tend to take vocal cues from the voice therapist or other individuals. The patient may consciously or unconsciously imitate a vocal pattern. The pattern may be appropriate to the therapist but inappropriate to the patient. The therapist must point out the vocal cues the patient is imitating as they occur and eliminate such vocal behavior. The patient must not become a vocal carbon copy of the therapist. He must be directed to the specific parameters of voice natural to him.

ILLUSTRATIVE THERAPY

Voice patients are notoriously unaware that other people have vocal symptoms and voice problems and that other patients have successfully undergone vocal therapy. Because of the lack of awareness of voice problems and vocal rehabilitation, it is often essential to bridge the gap of the new patient in voice therapy through direct contact with a former patient.

Illustrative therapy utilizes a former patient who has a similar problem, background, occupation, and personality to the new patient and who has resolved his voice problem. This former patient is brought into one therapy session to meet the new patient. The former patient relates his experience in vocal rehabilitation, the means of overcoming the voice problem, the frustrations involved in therapy, such as the maintenance and acceptance of the new voice, and the establishment of the automaticity of the new vocal pattern for all situations. This patient explains how his vocal symptoms and voice problem progressively disappeared during therapy and demonstrates the new voice compared to the old voice. The former patient also allows the new patient to hear tape recordings and Language Master cards of his old voice and the progression to his new voice. This type of approach is very reassuring to a new patient and allows the new patient to reaffirm the relevance and need for voice therapy.

The new patient needs a human contact, not just articles and books to recognize the voice problem. The fact that others have experienced voice problems and overcome them reassures the patient. A former patient who is a sales manager is more able to convey to a new patient, also a sales manager, the feasibility and appropriateness of vocal rehabilitation. Former patients are extremely cooperative in meeting with new voice patients, since the former patients are well aware of the confusion and disbelief they themselves had toward voice therapy when they first encountered it.

Before any illustrative therapy occurs the new patient is asked if he would like to meet with a former patient. A former patient is then sought who matches the new patient in his voice problem, personality, occupation, sex, and approximate age.

The therapist must use extreme caution and discretion with the selection of the former patient. The new patient may be adversely affected by the former patient's appearance, personality, comments, and especially the voice. If the former patient's voice, although appropriate to him, is displeasing to the new patient in pitch, tone focus, volume, and/or quality, this patient may elect to discontinue therapy.

Not all new voice patients elect to meet with a former voice patient. These new patients are convinced of the need for voice therapy by a strong physician referral or by their own recognition of the problem during the initial meeting. Sometimes a new patient elects to chat briefly with a former patient by telephone. Once again both patients are consulted for their approval prior to the conversation.

Another aspect of illustrative therapy is the use of tape replay to demonstrate before and after voices of former unidentified patients with similar dysphonias. Often this tape replay is sufficient to alleviate the new patient's anxieties concerning his voice problem and to increase his motivation to continue vocal rehabilitation. Illustrative therapy, while not necessary for all patients, is used for most patients in one form or another. Illustrative therapy, when needed, has proven to be a helpful and meaningful adjunct to modern vocal rehabilitation.

ASSOCIATE THERAPY

The most trying and difficult aspect of vocal rehabilitation for many patients is the carry-over of vocal training from the therapy session to outside situations. Since the carry-over is an essential element of vocal rehabilitation, it becomes vital to find a link or means of carry-over from the therapy session to the patient's everyday life. Associate therapy has been developed to meet this need. Associate therapy is that process whereby a wife or husband, friend, colleague, secretary, daughter, or son is brought into the therapy program in the initial stages of the rehabilitation program.

Associate therapy has been incorporated as an integral part of vocal rehabilitation because of comments and feelings of patients. They felt that their problem lacked understanding from others and that family members, friends, and colleagues failed to encourage or support their efforts in vocal rehabilitation. The failures that occurred because of this lack of support by relatives and friends required this additional concept not only to expedite therapy for all patients but also to assist those who were in need of additional support other than from the therapist.

Associate therapy has been found to be an effective and persuasive method for complimenting office therapy by allowing individuals who are close and meaningful to the patient to become part of the vocal rehabilitation program. Associate therapy meets the need of the patient and the process of carry-over in a fashion that encourages and solidifies the progress made during the therapy session.

Making close or meaningful relationships part of the rehabilitation program provides the patient with external support to buttress the internal insecurity that inevitably occurs and recurs during the vocal rehabilitation process. The patient is no longer isolated or alone in therapy. Others about him now assist him and allow him to assist himself more readily and easily.

In associate therapy the patient has an outside source or associate who can reassure him by reassessing his voice problem more objectively than the patient can himself. The therapist must decide during the initial contact with the associate, if he is capable of hearing the correct pitch level and tone focus in contrast to the incorrect pitch and tone focus. Surprisingly enough, nearly all associates, including secretaries, wives, husbands, and parents, have demonstrated an ability during the meeting with the therapist and patient to monitor the differences between the two voices. Even when the associate has a voice disorder himself, he is, nonetheless, usually able to help the patient. The voice patient also benefits from the open discussion of the voice problem, its causes, and its remedial variables.

With children, associate therapy must of necessity involve a parent, usually the mother. The child is not able to attend to the concepts of tone focus, pitch level, and breath support unless there is family understanding and support of the therapy afforded the child.

Associate therapy does not require repeated visits with the assistant, except in the case of children. Even with children, it is only some children who need repeated associate assistance in the office with the therapist consistently directing the parent for carry-over. With children, an older brother or sister may be of value to assist with the carry-over.

Occasionally in associate therapy, an assistant becomes a hazard or a hinderance, but this is of minor concern. One possible hazard is that the associate may minimize the difference between the old and new voices which confuses the patient. Another hazard occurs when the associate uses the patient's problem as a means of nagging and gnawing at the patient excessively or inappropriately. The associate must be able to monitor the patient's feeling state or, at least, the patient's ability to accept correction or suggestion at a particular time. If not, the carry-over procedure becomes a distasteful and disenchanting process.

When or if the associate therapy becomes more of a hinderance than a help, the associate is advised to cease affording assistance with the explanation that the patient is coming along nicely and can now sufficiently handle his own voice disorder by himself. The associate is also advised that vocal rehabilitation will be slowed down unless the patient is left to his own devices. He is told it is up to the patient himself to make the transition now that he is aware of what is needed in voice therapy.

Associate therapy is not a panacea, nor is it a means of assuring the success of vocal therapy. Associate therapy is simply an additional means of allowing for emotional support as well as affording carry-over in correct pitch level and tone focus in those cases where the associate has a good ear. Most patients who have been given associate therapy have benefited from the experience. Adults have reported that a family member or friend could subtly remind them of the correct pitch level during conversations or social events and thereby assist the patient. Although associate therapy may be used with most patients, it is not necessary nor feasible for all patients.

In summary, associate therapy affords basically two major benefits for the patient: (1) in most cases the associate can recognize the correct pitch and tone focus as contrasted to the old voice and assist the patient; and (2) the patient realizes that he is not alone or isolated and that others are aware of his problem and are willing to help him. Associate therapy affords both benefits to most patients.

BIBLIOTHERAPY

Patients need reading material relevant to their specific problems. Reprints of articles and portions of books written by the author are often used for patients in therapy. Reading material specific to each patient's voice disorder allows him a logical and dispassionate overview of the problem. The patient feels reassured from the written material that he is not alone in his voice disorder, and the material gives a reinforcement of the information provided in therapy. Of course, bibliotherapy is a supplement to therapy and must not be used as a substitute for therapy.

Chapters of books which may be helpful for bibliotherapy are Chapter VI in Anderson (1961), Chapter 7 in McClosky (1959), Chapters V and XIII in Brodnitz (1953), and Chapter XIII in Peacher (1966). For therapists who are interested in securing copies of specific articles written by this author for their own voice patients complimentary reprints are available.

GROUP VOICE THERAPY

Group voice therapy is useful for some patients. The group should consist of a limited number of patients who are in various stages of vocal rehabilitation. A group of all new patients does not function well because of their self-conscious attitudes and their lack of information and understanding of the problem. Patients in later stages of vocal rehabilitation work better together.

Group therapy in vocal rehabilitation differs from group therapy as practiced in the field of psychology. In psychology, there is discussion and group interaction for insight, understanding, and behavioral change. In vocal rehabilitation, there is discussion and some patient interaction, but more important, there must be practice on the various vocal elements to alter and improve the voice. The most important drawback to voice therapy in groups is that necessary practice or mechanical exercises to correct the vocal elements is almost impossible. Another drawback is the possibility of incompatible personalities which can impede vocal progress. Unlike other group therapy situations, personality alteration is not the primary concern.

The positive aspects of group voice therapy center around patient interaction and supportive therapy. Group voice therapy is based upon the premise that such a group can help to ventilate feelings, define the multiple causes that may have contributed to the onset and development of the respective voice problems, and gain insights in the culture and conditions that produced the voice disorder. Patients, finding that others in the group have similar or related symptoms, can openly discuss their voice problems and symptoms. The group experience affords the following: an emotional release, a catharsis of feeling for those patients able to speak out about their disorder; clarification of thinking about the problems and challenges involved in vocal therapy; understanding of the vocal image and vocal stereotypes; development of the new vocal identity; the realization that a new voice is relevant, needed, and appropriate, and is something to strive for, although the new voice sounds strange and disenchanting to the patient. Those who are completing therapy are able to reassure those who are entering therapy of the point and purpose of therapy and are able to demonstrate their progress to the newcomer.

The negative aspects of group therapy at this point outweigh the positive aspects. When patients are referred for voice therapy, they are queasy and self-conscious about their voices and voice therapy. These patients often do not take kindly to vocal analysis in groups. From clinical experience in vocal rehabilitation, lower economic status patients have been willing to work in a group only because of the low fee charged for group therapy; the higher economic status patients have usually declined group therapy.

From the author's own experience as a student in classes of

voice training and from reviewing such experiences with other students, confusion and disappointment have been the net result. The development of one's own voice and vocal potential was often not completed. Group therapy also does not allow for as much individual attention and practice of the vocal variables. Each patient wants and needs individual practice for his specific voice, location and maintenance of the optimal pitch level, and so on. Group voice therapy may involve a protracted period of time for completion of therapy because of the lack of practice time and individual guidance.

Another major problem involves the time scheduling for groups. Because of this scheduling problem, different types of voice problems and divergent personalities may be placed in the same group, whereas group therapy should have homogenous voice problems and flexible personalities. Otherwise, therapy is disruptive and inefficient.

Group voice therapy may be successful in an ideal situation. This would occur if the members of the group were within a workable age span, if the voice problems were essentially alike, if there were a mixture of old and new patients, and if the personalities within the group were compatible. Group therapy for vocal psychotherapy can be very helpful because of insights and understanding gained through discussion of the vocal image and vocal identity; however, this is only one part of vocal rehabilitation.

Group voice therapy may serve as an adjunct to individual vocal rehabilitation and may be utilized for one session or for a limited number of sessions to take advantage of the positive aspects of group therapy. On the whole, group voice therapy has not been too successful or meaningful for those involved in it. More research is needed to determine the effectiveness of group therapy for vocal problems.

PART 3
VOCAL REHABILITATION:
PROCESS AND PROBLEMS

RELATED ASPECTS OF VOCAL REHABILITATION
Art of the Therapist

The method of vocal rehabilitation, whether traditional or modern, is usually as effective as the person using it. The method alone is not the deciding factor. The therapist must always be cognizant of the pitfalls of this method or any method he is using. A competent voice therapist may be successful with many methods. A competent voice therapist is one who can analyze a voice into its component aspects, define any deviant attributes, and provide a meaningful program of vocal therapy that eliminates negative vocal symptoms and produces an efficient and/or artistic voice. Moore (1971, p. 5) writes: "An awareness of the audible components of vocal sound and the development of the capacity to recognize them are essential to successful management of voice disorders."*

A competent voice therapist must be aware, however, that therapy is based not only upon the science or techniques of vocal rehabilitation but also upon the art of vocal rehabilitation. The therapist must remember that he is treating the whole person, not just the voice problem. Although the therapist must know and competently practice vocal rehabilitation techniques, technical vocal guidance alone is not sufficient. The therapist must be aware of the patient's feeling state and level of understanding; he must treat the patient in regard to that reality. The science without the art does not allow for meaningful therapy.

Meaningful therapy occurs only through the rapport and relatedness of the two individuals, patient and therapist. Rapport, an integral factor in vocal rehabilitation, may be established in various ways, such as being a good listener, finding common grounds of interest, background, or experience, and being sensitive to the patient's needs. Vocal therapy succeeds only when the patient relates to the therapist, has confidence and faith in the

---

* G. Paul Moore, *Organic Voice Disorders,* p. 5. Copyright 1971, Prentice-Hall, Englewood Cliffs, New Jersey.

therapist, and realizes that the therapist is competent and able to help him. Some patients have made comments such as "Were it not for your understanding and encouragement I would not have continued." Other patients have indicated a sense of humor is needed.

Voice therapy may be accepted or declined because of the personality of the therapist. Clinical experience reveals that the patients are very concerned with the personality of the therapist. The therapist must be sensitive to the specific needs, desires, hopes, and demands of the patient insofar as vocal rehabilitation is concerned. He cannot insist that the patient adjust to him during therapy. The therapist's personality and his ability to be flexible enough to meet the needs and demands of the patient's personality to a reasonable degree is essential.

The therapist must be congruent and authentic to himself and to his patients in the therapy situation. He must have the type of personality that conveys to the patient his genuine interest and concern for the patient. The therapist needs warmth, sincerity, understanding, perception, and patience. He also needs freshness and strength of mind and body in order to keep his enthusiasm, stimulability, and positive attitude during therapy. The personality of the therapist can make or break vocal rehabilitation. Therapy, especially voice therapy, is not an impersonal affair.

During the course of vocal rehabilitation, transference may occur. Transference is a carry-over by the patient of his feelings, emotions, and reactions to the therapist and to the therapeutic situation. This is due to the therapist's personality and behavior which reminds the patient of past and present relationships, such as those with family members or associates. Transference may have either a positive or a negative effect. If the transferred feelings and reactions are negative, the patient may express hostility and aggression toward the therapist. The therapist must be aware of and recognize the process of transference in voice patients. By understanding transference, the therapist may use this natural feeling state to assist the patient in overcoming the voice problem. It is seldom relevant to discuss the transference condition with the patient, except in situations in which there is a highly negative reaction.

The matter of countertransference should also be considered. The therapist may project his feelings and emotions toward the patient because the patient reminds the therapist of past or present associations. Cognizance and understanding of this feeling state is essential for the therapist in order to afford and to facilitate therapy.

The approach for all patients is similar yet different. The therapist must always find out what the patient needs and wants from the therapist in the way of a relationship in vocal rehabilitation. The relationship at first may be more important than the vocal assistance rendered to the patient.

A few patients have had negative experiences regarding therapy or treatment in another discipline. This type of patient may be skeptical of the voice therapist who also offers a type of therapy. It is necessary to uncover the relevant negative factors and feelings the patient has that can affect vocal rehabilitation.

The voice therapist must be aware that initially the patient may be doubtful and uncomfortable in vocal rehabilitation. Training the speaking voice is an unheard of and strange situation for nearly all voice patients. The therapist must be able to accept these uncertainties of the patient and convince the patient that voice therapy is relevant and essential. He must often reassure the patient that his voice problem is not singular nor unique, that many others have experienced similar voice disorders, and that most patients overcome their voice problems.

The therapist must anticipate problems in therapy. For instance, after establishing the optimal pitch level, there will often be tension underneath the mandible and within the soft palate. These few positive vocal symptoms may frighten the patient into discontinuing the new pitch given to him. The therapist must reassure the patient before these symptoms ever occur that they will occur and also that they will disappear quite soon.

The therapist must understand that the patient's personality and his threshold of pain determine his physical and psychological reactions to the voice disorder. Two patients may have similar voice disorders, but their reactions may be dissimilar. The therapist must be aware of these variables and work within their confines.

The art of the therapist must take into account the personality of the patient and his drive to overcome the voice problem. He must allow those patients who insist upon their own vocal rehabilitation path to pursue it until they clearly understand that their way will not achieve success. For example, the need to move from work on the pitch level to breathing should be based upon the patient's ability to produce the correct pitch consistently and easily; however, some patients insist upon moving quickly to breath support before they have mastered the correct pitch level. Although nearly all of these patients fail in this venture, it may be necessary to allow them their failure, or else they believe that the therapist is proceeding too slowly in therapy. When the patient is unable to keep his correct pitch while practicing breath support, he is more willing to heed the directions of the voice therapist.

The therapist must work with each patient at the rate in which the patient is able to progress and feels most comfortable. If the therapy is too slow, the patient may discontinue for lack of progress and for continuation of vocal symptoms. If therapy is too fast, the patient may be unable to integrate the new motor patterns and vocal habits into his daily activities and therefore experience marked frustration and repeated failure. The amount of pressure, internal and external, that the patient can bear must be gauged by the therapist so that vocal rehabilitation proceeds as comfortably, as purposefully, yet as quickly as possible.

The art of the therapist must rely upon the therapist's discretion and judgement, which is based upon his interpretation and understanding of the patient's feelings and thoughts. For instance, illustrative therapy usually occurs early in vocal rehabilitation, but the therapist may decide the patient needs this type of assistance at any stage of therapy.

Vocal rehabilitation is a laborious process. There are elements within it, such as changing the pitch level, adjusting to a new tone focus, establishing correct breath support, which require mechanical practice at the Language Master. If the patient is allowed to remain with these exercises, he may become bored with the practice and disinterested in the process. To add variety and interest, the therapist must alternate practice at the Language

Master with conversation. The patient is also able to talk about his ability or disability in performing the mechanical exercises. As the mechanical aspects of therapy are mastered, there is a greater opportunity for conversation and an overview of the elements which have and do continue to contribute to the voice disorder, such as the vocal image and its attendant emotional or physical problems.

The voice therapist must have sufficient knowledge to be able to answer the patients' questions concerning voice and vocal rehabilitation. A patient may have a number of questions he wants to ask, but he may feel constrained or hesitant to do so in the fear that he is being unreasonable in asking questions. He may be afraid that he is interfering with his therapy or that he is slowing down the therapy process. Other patients hesitate to ask questions regarding vocal symptoms because they fear they are exposing themselves as being abnormal in disclosing their symptoms, feelings, and thoughts. By asking questions, the patient is emotionally and intellectually stripping himself and must be helped to view his voice problem clearly and without emotion. Patients must be reassured that all questions are entirely proper, normal, desirable, and facilitative to the process of therapy. Questions are a form of catharsis, a type of vocal psychotherapy. By answering a patient's questions comfortably and easily, the patient is reassured and further rapport is established. The patient quickly loses confidence in a therapist who cannot answer his questions meaningfully and directly.

The therapist's personality, which must secure empathy, rapport, and motivation from the voice patient, is a major factor in the art of voice therapy. The art of the therapist is to determine what each patient needs from him, when, why, and how; however, unless the therapist has authentic knowledge of the science of vocal rehabilitation, the process itself will fail and the problems of the voice disorder will continue.

Initial Evaluation

The initial evaluation is one of the most significant encounters between the patient and the therapist. What the therapist says and does purposefully or unintentionally affects the patient.

The therapist's grasp of the patient's problem, needs, and feeling state toward the voice disorder determines the course of therapy. The evaluation may appear to be a routine procedure to the patient, but it should be far more than that to the therapist. The patient is reassured by the therapist's manner and method that his problem is not unique nor uncommon. The patient may enter therapy with full confidence or decline to enter therapy on the basis of the initial contact with the therapist, which is usually the evaluation. This evaluation sets the stage for the rapport between patient and therapist.

The patient and the therapist fill out an evaluation form (see Appendix A). The patient is assured by the therapist that all information written on forms or recorded on tape is confidential. The patient is next given a check sheet of negative sensory and auditory vocal symptoms (see Appendix B). The patient indicates which of these symptoms he is experiencing at this time. The patient is directed to modify or alter the wording of any symptom so that it applies specifically to his case. For example, the symptom sheet lists "Clear voice in the morning with tired or foggy voice in the afternoon or evening." A patient may experience the reverse of this condition. By determining the number of symptoms and the extent of each symptom, the therapist can deduce the degree of the problem, acute or chronic. The symptom sheet is reviewed periodically and at the termination of therapy.

The next procedure is to make a master tape by recording the patient's voice on a high fidelity tape recorder, such as the Tandberg®. This master tape recording consists of an interview with the patient regarding his voice problem: the length of time he has had the problem; the type of problem he has; the symptoms he is experiencing from his voice disorder; contributory factors to the voice disorder, such as smoking, sinusitis, postnasal drip, medication, and hormones; surgeries; emotional or physical problems which may affect the voice; the presence of the vocal image; and any other specific aspects which may be pertinent to that particular individual. The patient's name and the date is recorded at the beginning and at the end of the tape recording. The patient must be recorded for a sufficient amount of time so as to allow for superimposition of the new voice upon the original tape at a later date.

The patient also records on one track of several Language Master cards. On one card, he gives his name and the date. On a series of cards, the patient counts to fifteen and describes his vocal symptoms and his voice problem.

The location of the optimal pitch level and the proper tone focus is determined during this initial meeting, unless the patient is severely dysphonic (a situation previously discussed). The patient is directed to the new pitch and tone focus which is usually recorded on one track of several Language Master cards.

The patient is given the opportunity to listen to his old voice. The patient is asked, "Do you want to hear how you sound? It would be helpful for you to hear your own voice." (Only a miniscule number of patients have declined to listen to their own voices.) The patient may also listen to the new voice. His reaction to the old voice and to the new voice is briefly reviewed by the therapist, who outlines the influence of the old vocal image when it is applicable and discusses the new vocal image which the patient will develop. Further discussion of contributory factors to the voice disorder may be necessary, such as physical or emotional trauma, poor vocal habits, lack of vocal training, and inadequate vocal models. Other discussion may include the relationship of the morning voice and the basal pitch to the new voice and the new positive vocal symptoms the patient may experience from using the new pitch.

The therapist must be aware that a few patients use an optimal pitch level during the initial evaluation. However, when they are functioning in their professional capacity, such as a teacher, a newscaster, a trial lawyer, or when they are under pressure, they drop several tones below the optimal pitch level. During the evaluation or in therapy, they apparently do not feel pressured or feel they have to maintain a vocal image.

The patient must be reassured throughout the evaluation that he is not unusual in experiencing a voice disorder and that he can overcome this disorder through vocal rehabilitation. Before and after tapes of previous patients are played for him. (Patient names and identification are eliminated. Any well-known personality who could be identified by voice alone is never used.) The patient is given reprints of articles to read which are applicable to his specific type of voice disorder. (The articles are discussed in the next session if the patient desires.) The patient is given suggestions for good vocal hygiene which are also afforded him in some of the reprints.

The patient must be convinced of the relevance of vocal rehabilitation to his specific voice problem. If the therapist feels that illustrative therapy would be helpful, the patient is asked if he would like to meet a patient in the next session who has completed vocal rehabilitation or even talk to a former patient by phone in the initial evaluation. The patient is also offered the opportunity for associate therapy by bringing someone to the next session.

The prognosis is discussed during this initial session; however, no guarantees should be given regarding the duration of therapy or the outcome of therapy. The patient is given exercises to practice between sessions, and a practice routine is suggested. The patient and the therapist decide upon the frequency of the therapy sessions and set up a program of therapy.

When the patient is a child, the parents are usually present during the initial evaluation and may assist the child in answering questions. If the patient is an adolescent, the parents may or may not be present, depending upon the individual patient. The mother is usually the parental figure who brings the child to therapy and assists the child at home. If the parent is not present, she is brought in at the close of the session. At this time, the therapist discusses the voice disorder as well as the causes and contributory factors of the disorder. The parent hears the old and new voices, is told the extent and duration of practice, and is given reprints to read. The therapist answers any questions the parent may have. The prognosis as well as the frequency of meetings is reviewed. The initial evaluation for the adolescent is similar to that for the adult.

Preferably before the initial interview and always prior to the initiation of vocal rehabilitation, the dysphonic person should have a laryngeal examination by a laryngologist. This examination must be current. If the patient is beginning vocal rehabilitation, the laryngologist should afford the voice therapist an initial report by letter or by telephone of the condition of the vocal folds and larynx. If possible, a written report including a diagrammatic sketch of the vocal folds showing lesions, paralysis, or other conditions should be made by the laryngologist and sent to the voice therapist.

Frequency and Duration of Therapy

The frequency of therapy for voice cases is determined by the patient's needs and demands and the therapist's evaluation and decision of what is best for the patient. Initially, the patient should be seen two or three times weekly until he can control the correct pitch level, tone focus, and breath support automatically, utilizing them within the therapy session and outside the office. This ideal approach affords the best and the fastest results.

The frequency of therapy sessions moves from two or three weekly meetings to twice weekly to once weekly. As the patient masters the various elements of voice, the patient and the therapist agreeing upon the patient's progress, the frequency is reduced to once every two weeks for a few sessions, then to once a month, and finally to once every three months. By this system of diminished frequency, the patient is able to determine his ability to control his voice and the extent of his vocal recovery.

Patients who wish to hasten the vocal rehabilitative process are afforded intensive therapy. Intensive vocal rehabilitation may be defined as one to six sessions daily from one to six weeks. This type of therapy is requested by the patient. Usually these patients are in a hurry to overcome their vocal problem for one reason or another. They are executives, top salesmen, or TV and film personalities who may have only a brief period of time to overcome the voice problem. Other patients may come from distant places specifically for vocal rehabilitation and are able to remain in the area only for a short period of time.

The duration of therapy is related to the frequency of therapy, to the severity of the problem, to the patient's motivation and cooperation, to the patient's ability to monitor his voice and to reevaluate his old voice as compared to the new voice, to the extent and degree of the vocal image involved, and to the patient's ego strength to confront the old vocal image and accept the new vocal image. The duration of therapy is also dependent upon the therapist's ability to relate to the patient, the therapist's competence in determining and directing the patient to the optimal pitch level and to the correct tone focus, the therapist's skill in demonstrating a correct and incorrect pitch level, tone focus, and breath support, and his ability to serve as a voice model for the patient. The faster the correct pitch level is determined and utilized, causing an alleviation and/or elimination of vocal symptoms, the more responsive will be the patient who gains additional confidence in the therapist and more acceptance of therapy. This, in turn, speeds up the therapy process.

Most patients with functional misphonia require one to six months of vocal rehabilitation. This is considered short-term therapy. Some of these patients are able to resolve their voice disorders within one month; approximately 20 percent of those with functional misphonia who completed therapy did so in one month. The majority of patients require three to six months. A limited number of patients require six to twelve months or more (long-term therapy). Of those patients with functional misphonia, 83.1 percent needed short-term therapy (six months or less) and 16.9 percent required long-term therapy (over six months).

Special Needs

Patients seek specific vocal fulfillment in voice therapy. Most patients want an elimination of symptoms, such as hoarseness or vocal fatigue, while others are concerned with obtaining a good carrying voice. The patient may want to speak continuously without vocal fatigue and with a good flexible tone that is expressive of his personality.

Some individuals have to talk in and over noise since they are workers or supervisors in that type of environment. Actors, lawyers, and teachers have need for volume as they speak to large audiences. These individuals must be afforded: (1) an optimal pitch level; (2) marked control of the proper tone focus; (3)

oronasopharyngeal resonance with heightened nasal resonance (precluding nasality); and (4) midsection breath support. When the patient has mastered the coordination of these factors, the voice carries over the noise. This nonpathological voice with carrying power is termed a "projected voice." Without midsection breath support laryngeal and pharyngeal tensions will occur. Some children must be taught how to project the voice or else they will continually shout. Shouting is the use of excessive volume, stress upon laryngopharyngeal resonance, an incorrect pitch level, and upper chest or clavicular breath support.

Patients should not change occupations because of voice problems. Following vocal rehabilitation, a patient should be able to use his voice as much as is necessary in his job. If the person must yell or talk above noise in his job, he is taught how to project his voice so that he does not shout and injure his larynx.

Some individuals earn their living by telephone activities. Telephone operators, salespeople, and stockbrokers belong in this category. These individuals need a durable, pleasant voice. They have a marked tendency to use the intimate or confidential telephone voice. They fail to realize that they could use an intimate or confidential voice that is equally agreeable and saleable by keeping the pitch range optimal and the volume moderate.

Efficient Voice

The efficient voice would be defined as a functional voice which affords the maximum amount of sound and degree of usage with a minimum amount of effort and which has an aesthetic acceptance by listeners. Van Wye (1936, p. 644) has defined the efficient voice:

> The efficient voice in speech is one that does the work allotted to it—just as any other efficient mechanism does its work—with a maximum of effect, a wise conservation of energy, and a large degree of esthetic gratification.

Anderson (1961, pp. 18-19) writes:

> Voice production should be as simple and effortless as possible. No great amount of energy should be required to produce a vocal tone even of considerable loudness, nor should the vocal organs become fatigued or irritated even after prolonged, steady use under normal

conditions. Ordinarily there should be no feeling of strain or tension in the throat during vocalization.

Most patients want a functional and efficient voice, not an artistic voice. They want to overcome the voice disorder and secure a comfortable, durable and natural voice without negative vocal symptoms. They have neither the time nor the interest to seek an artistic voice.

The establishment of an efficient voice in the overwhelming number of voice cases requires an elevated pitch level and a new tone focus. Holmes (1931, p. 236) writes: "Efficient voice production cannot be achieved unless 'frontal placement' is established." Quite often the tone focus is essentially within the laryngopharynx. The new tone focus must emphasize oronasal resonance blended within the voice so that nasality does not occur. Use of the optimal pitch level also affords greater intelligibility of speech.

The so-called normal voice, which is used by the majority of the population, is usually not an efficient voice. Unfortunately, most individuals are unaware that the normal voice may be an inefficient voice. Van Wye (1936) remarks that 99 out of 100 voices do not meet his criteria for an efficient voice.

The individual with a normal voice may experience any number of negative vocal symptoms, but he may not realize their significance. Also, two individuals may react differently to similar symptoms. One individual who has inflamed vocal folds and throat tension during speaking may not be incapacitated or disabled in speech or in personality effect. Another individual with the same problem may be severely affected by such symptoms in speech as well as in personality. The reaction to the vocal symptoms and the effect upon communication and personality are essentially the factors that determine the severity of the voice disorder and the inefficiency of the voice from the *individual's* point of view.

Time and place are determining factors in the aesthetic acceptance or nonacceptance of the "normal" voice. In some parts of the United States, a nasal voice might be acceptable to its listeners. The nasal twang or hillbilly voice is usually pitched above the optimal level and contains an excessive amount of nasopharyngeal resonance. This voice may be considered efficient in terms of carrying power and ease of projection, but it is aesthetically unfulfilling to listeners outside of the cultural setting in which it may prevail.

The question of efficiency or inefficiency in voice must ultimately rest with *both* the patient and the voice therapist. The patient is usually able to determine the inefficiency of voice once the negative vocal symptoms are clearly pointed out to him. The patient must realize that inflamed or swollen vocal folds during or after speaking, functional bowed vocal folds, nodes, polyps, contact ulcers, and possibly other growths upon the vocal folds are due to inefficient use of the voice. When the patient is made aware of sensory symptoms that indicate vocal misuse or abuse, he becomes cognizant of the extent and degree of his inefficient voice. The patient must be alerted to the auditory symptoms by tape replay so that he is able to determine the extent of vocal impairment relating to pitch, tone focus, quality, volume, and rate. The therapist and the patient together determine the extent and degree of the inefficient voice. The voice therapist, then, advises the patient as to the changes needed for the patient to acquire an efficient voice.

Artistic Voice

An artistic voice is one which can be classified as efficient in producing the greatest amount of sound for the least amount of effort, which sounds aesthetic, which is natural to the speaker's vocal abilities, and which reaches the individual's fullest vocal potential. An efficient voice is often not an artistic voice. Both voices have a balanced oral and nasal resonance and an optimal pitch level. The artistic voice is more concerned with the ultimate development of a graceful and flexible voice utilizing the total pitch range, which is coordinated with precise midsection breath support. In defining the goal of therapy, Brodnitz (1963, p. 151) states:

> In the functional disorders the therapy aims at the restoration of a voice that is well produced, stands up under prolonged use, and serves satisfactorily as an instrument of communication and of professional or artistic use.

Individuals in TV, radio, movies and stage feel the need to have a low-pitched voice for professional work (Cooper, 1970l). At the beginning of vocal rehabilitation, when they first hear the new voice, they often feel that the optimal pitch is not low enough for this type of work. These individuals are directed by the voice therapist to use the optimal pitch outside of professional activities and the low-pitched voice during professional activities, if they so insist. In this manner they use a put-on voice for professional purposes, realize it, and alter the vocal pattern as soon as they can. Most broadcasters, actors, and actresses desire to develop their real voice, but they prefer to make the change-over from the old to the new voice gradually so that it will not be noticed by their audiences. When the voice change is completed, these individuals report that no one seems to realize the voice has changed at all, though to themselves they have changed noticeably in pitch, tone focus, and quality of voice. They have now developed an artistic voice which is the ability to use their voice in the best possible way in pitch, tone focus, quality, breath support, volume, and rate (Cooper, 1970j). When the artistic voice is mastered, the low-pitched put-on voice is no longer needed or used.

Singing and Voice Disorders

Voice disorders in singers may be caused by vocal misuse of the singing voice or vocal misuse of the speaking voice. Vocal misuse initially of either the speaking voice or the singing voice may lead eventually to misuse of the other voice. Singers who have been seen in vocal rehabilitation have been misusing the speaking voice in all cases and misusing the singing voice in some cases.

Cooper (1970i, p. 53) comments:

> The singing and speaking voices should have basically the same pitch level and range and tone focus. A marked difference between the singing and speaking voices should alert the individual to the fact that one of the two voices is not being used properly.

In most singers who have been seen in vocal rehabilitation, the speaking voice was too low in pitch.

Negative vocal symptoms in either the speaking or the singing voice should not be considered normal. These negative vocal symptoms are often caused by incorrect vocal habits, poor vocal hygiene, lack of or poor vocal training, imitation, or the vocal image. Cooper (1970i, p. 53) has found:

> Amateur singers frequently do not sing in the proper range, either because they are unaware of their optimal pitch range or because they are assigned incorrect pitch ranges to use in group singing.

He (1970c, p. 7) also comments:

> Singers are often oblivious to good vocal hygiene. They talk many hours a day in adverse circumstances (yelling in cars, talking above noise at rehearsal or at parties) and irritate the vocal cords before they arrive for the presentation.

Voorhees (1914, p. 342) comments: "Flatau believes that 80 per cent of all young singers are affected by phonasthenia by the end of their third year of study." According to Greene (1968, p. 1150):

> The great majority of ordinary singers whether professional or amateur are imperfectly trained by teachers of singing who have often drifted into their teaching responsibilities by way of piano or organ playing and a love of music and singing.

Imitation and the vocal image exist in singing as well as in speaking. Cooper (1970i, p. 53) discusses this problem:

> In singing, too, various vocal styles and ranges may well influence a singer to adopt a range and style unsuitable for his vocal abilities. A singer, for example, might strive to sound like someone he admires.

Singers with functional or organic dysphonias are given vocal rehabilitation primarily for the speaking voice and secondarily for the singing voice. Vocal rehabilitation is as applicable for the singing voice as it is for the speaking voice, since misuse of one voice affects the other voice. Singers, in general, have an excellent prognosis in vocal rehabilitation.

Vocal Hygiene

A program of good vocal hygiene must be integrated within the total program of vocal rehabilitation. Relative to the patient and the circumstances, some of the suggestions which are given to patients are as follows:

1. Use moderate volume throughout the day in all situations.

2. Avoid talking in noisy situations, such as in any form of transportation (trains, planes, cars, buses, and subways), in factories, or at construction sites.

3. Avoid competing with loud conversation at a party, gathering, or conference.

4. Avoid talking under or over music or sound from a television set, radio, record player, or tape recorder.

5. Do not shout or yell in any situations, including ball games, at school, with family members, and during recreational activities (bowling, tennis, swimming).

6. Do not sing in groups. Do not sing solo if untrained.

7. Try to avoid or minimize any violent disturbances of the vocal folds, such as coughing, clearing the throat, sneezing, crying, and laughing.

8. Avoid any strenuous exercise, such as lifting, pushing, or pulling (for contact ulcer patients).

9. Generally curtail smoking and drinking, if excessive.

10. Avoid vocal rest, unless specifically ordered by the laryngologist or voice therapist.

11. Continue *maximum* use of the speaking voice, with moderate volume.

12. Maintain an optimal pitch level with moderate volume when experiencing a cold or upper respiratory infection. Do not pamper the voice by talking under the cold.

Vocal hygiene is an individual matter. Some patients require a longer period of time for vocal rest following surgery than other patients. Some women are able to talk in a noisy atmosphere without ill effect to the voice because the pitch of the voice is high enough to afford carrying power without undue effort. General rules of good vocal hygiene are given to all patients, but the therapist and patient must interpret these suggestions to fit the patient's individual needs and voice.

Vocal Mythology

Vocal mythology is a major consideration in vocal rehabilitation. Vocal mythology encompasses common beliefs held by most individuals regarding the voice, vocal usage, causes for voice problems, and treatment for voice disorders. As the name implies, vocal mythology espouses a number of unfounded assumptions and presumptions which are fundamentally incorrect and untrue. Vocal mythology includes beliefs which create vocal stereotypes and vocal images.

Some beliefs revolve around vocal usage. Many believe that a tired voice is natural or normal following brief or prolonged speaking. These people expect the muscles of the voice (laryngeal and pharyngeal muscles) to tire. They accept the hoarseness, the fatigue of voice, and the additional effort required to produce voice as being normal. They may also believe that overuse of the voice causes a voice problem, a tired voice, hoarseness, or laryngitis. Overuse is a nebulous term defined by some as an hour or so of talking and by others as an extended period of time involving three to eight hours. These same individuals may believe that some people are born with a weak throat or voice and that they will always experience difficulty with the voice.

These are myths because the well-used voice does not tire, does not produce negative vocal symptoms, and does not require additional effort to speak. Overuse per se does not create voice problems; misuse and abuse of the voice create the problems. Any use of a misused and abused voice may cause a voice disorder. The efficient or well-produced voice may be used indefinitely as long as the individual is not fatigued and is in good health. Persons with "weak throats" have not been found in clinical voice therapy.

Vocal mythology includes irrelevant suggestions for treatment of a voice problem. Some people try gargles, milk and honey, hot tea and lemon, throat sprays, pills, steam, and vitamins, among other remedies. These methods are in part palliative not curative. Some of them may be helpful for limited periods of time. However, they merely mask the symptoms; they do not remove the cause which is usually vocal misuse and abuse. Other myths are to stop talking or limit the talking and observe vocal rest, a change of occupation if talking is required in the present one, and learning to relax and to be calm. Some of these suggestions are unrealistic if not impossible. Job change is simply not feasible; vocal rest for any extended period of time is unreasonable. A person cannot relax simply because he knows he should, and tranquilizers cannot be provided permanently.

Individuals may have myths about vocal rehabilitation. Some patients believe that they cannot be helped by vocal rehabilitation. They express the view that good voices are born, that you either have a good voice or you don't. They do not feel that good voices can be developed. Others think they cannot be helped because they have a "tin ear" or an inability to distinguish different pitches. Still others are of the opinion that vocal rehabilitation is voice training for actors, actresses, newscasters —those who require an aesthetically professional speaking voice. Another myth is that voice training is for the singing voice only.

Vocal rehabilitation is applicable and meaningful to any individual who encounters negative vocal symptoms, especially for one who has a need to use the speaking voice routinely and repeatedly to fulfill either his job or his personality. Efficient and superior voices are developed, as is the ability to hear and maintain the optimal pitch.

Another vocal myth is that one or two sessions of vocal therapy will provide sufficient insight, guidance, and improvement for the misused voice. While 10 percent of about 1406 patients have overcome the voice problem within one month of therapy, most patients require three months to one year. Another myth is that hypnotism can eliminate the voice problem. While hypnotism is of value for some disorders and problems, its relevance to vocal rehabilitation remains nil.

A vocal myth that has been encountered in vocal rehabilitation is that the tongue must be able to perform certain acrobatic movements in order to improve the voice. This tongue in cheek technique does not appear to have much relevance other than the fact that it keeps one's tongue wagging.

Other myths concern breathing. Some believe that one must take a deep breath in order to speak, and in taking this deep breath, the chest should expand. In reality, only a small intake of air is necessary for speech if the exhalation is controlled. The chest should not heave in inhalation or in exhalation.

Other therapists may encounter additional myths regarding the voice. The sophisticated voice therapist can underscore fact from fiction and vocal truth from vocal mythology.

FACTORS INFLUENCING PROGRESS IN VOCAL REHABILITATION

The first factor is acceptability of the problem and acceptability of vocal rehabilitation as a means of resolving the voice problem. Most people have never heard of vocal rehabilitation. The inability of some patients to accept their voice problem and vocal rehabilitation leads to a continued vocal neurosis and vocal pathology. Vocal rehabilitation often confronts a vocal cultural lag; society is unaware of vocal rehabilitation. Voice problems are unreal and unnatural. As one patient said, "People aren't convinced that it is a real problem when you lose your voice or have a voice difficulty."

A strong medical referral from a physician in whom the patient believes greatly influences acceptability. Medical practitioners, even laryngologists, may be unsophisticated regarding vocal rehabilitation for functional voice disorders, particularly functional misphonia. When feasible, the voice therapist can discuss with the physician the process and extent of vocal rehabilitation. Otherwise, the physician may tell the patient that only a single session is necessary and that the voice therapist will give the patient hints for changing his voice in this session, which the voice therapist cannot do. When the patient learns the length of time required for vocal rehabilitation and what is involved after expecting one session, the patient, the physician, and the voice therapist are dissatisfied and unhappy.

In addition to a strong physician referral, other methods of establishing the acceptability have been previously discussed in other sections and are summarized as follows: (1) Acceptance of the voice therapist. The patient accepts the voice therapist's opinion and evaluation. (2) Negative vocal symptoms. From the list of negative vocal symptoms, the patient realizes he is experiencing relevant ones. (3) Tapes of patients' voices before and after vocal rehabilitation. The patient is able to hear the contrast between before and after voices of other patients who have had voice disorders. (4) Location of the patient's optimal pitch level and tone focus. The patient is able to hear the difference between his habitual voice and his optimal pitch and proper tone focus. (5) Bibliotherapy. The patient accepts the voice disorder and its cause(s) from reading relevant articles and/or books. (6) Illustrative therapy. The new patient is convinced by a former patient who has overcome his voice disorder. (7) Associate therapy. A close relative or friend of the patient acts as an independent judge to assist the patient in accepting his voice disorder and his new voice. All of these possibilities are not used with every patient. The voice therapist must decide which are relevant to the patient's needs.

Motivation is another factor influencing progress. Motivation comes not only from the patient but also inherently from everything the voice therapist says and does. The patient must be motivated to deal with and overcome his voice disorders. The greater the degree of motivation there is, the faster his rate of vocal recovery will be. This, of course, presupposes that the voice therapist is competent and that his enthusiasm and belief in vocal rehabilitation is embedded in successful experiences with voice disorders.

A few patients are motivated by a realistic fear that continued misuse will result in a malignant condition of the vocal folds. Some patients are motivated by the possible need of surgery or by surgery itself. Other patients are fearful that the negative vocal symptoms will further expand to include additional symptoms and the intensity and frequency of the discomfort will increase. Most patients are motivated by the desire to relieve and end the symptoms. The earlier these symptoms are attended to, the greater the motivation of the patient will be, not only to continue therapy but also to pursue all directions offered him in therapy.

Patients vary in the type, number, duration, and severity of negative vocal symptoms as well as in the concern for the symptoms which they present. One patient's need to remove a sore throat may be the motivating factor for vocal rehabilitation. The improved voice may be appreciated later, but removal of the sore throat is a basic and overriding concern to the patient at present. Another patient may be concerned with general symptom removal. Again, this patient is concerned with voice improvement only insomuch as this improvement removes the negative vocal symptoms. Improving the speaking voice and making it clearer and better able to respond to speaking conditions and demands may be of minor consideration to these patients.

The therapist must ascertain the patient's hierarchy of negative vocal symptoms. Once the therapist determines which of the negative vocal symptoms is most important for the patient to eliminate, he is able to reassure the patient that this symptom will be alleviated and removed through one or more of the various aspects of vocal rehabilitation. Specific symptom removal becomes the goal of this patient rather than general voice improvement, which is not his concern.

In other patients, motivation comes from the hope that the vocal problem can be resolved. If the hope remains only a hope in that the voice does not improve and the vocal symptoms are not eliminated within a reasonable period of time, the patient loses his motivation to continue therapy or to give his utmost in therapy. Motivation may initially come from outside sources, but these outside sources give way to internal motivation when the symptoms are being eliminated.

SIGNS OF PROGRESS IN VOCAL REHABILITATION

The elimination of the negative vocal symptoms indexes the extent of vocal rehabilitation progress and success. The patient initially indicates the negative sensory and auditory vocal symptoms by checking them off on a symptom sheet and by describing the symptoms on the original tape. A superimposition at a later date upon the original tape recording reveals the auditory degree of vocal improvement. The patient is able to judge for himself the positive change in the listenability of his voice. The sensory progress is detected when the patient experiences durability, comfort, and flexibility of his voice in all normal speaking situations throughout the day. Periodic examinations and reports by the laryngologist are necessary as the patient is undergoing therapy and a final examination after the patient has completed vocal rehabilitation. These periodic and final reports are compared with the initial report for evidence of the patient's progress in eliminating visual symptoms.

All patients in voice therapy need constant reassurance about their training and their progress. This must not be a blatant assurance given too often but a sincere reassurance that allows the patient to move forward. Unless patients know they are moving ahead, they are subject to their own doubts and to the doubts of others who find fault and discourage training the speaking voice. The patient always needs encouragement and support for his successes as well as understanding and acceptance for his failures.

Instructions, directions, and explanations must be repeated again and again by the voice therapist at the beginning of therapy and during therapy until the patient digests and comprehends the information. When the patient realizes the therapist is repetitive, the patient is improving because he is absorbing, understanding, and remembering the material.

Before the patient improves during vocal rehabilitation, he often becomes worse temporarily as positive vocal symptoms appear. Initially he is told that new kinesthetic symptoms, such as tension and/or acute pain, will occur underneath the mandible and at the back of the throat. For most patients the new positive vocal symptoms move from the lower laryngopharynx and center under the mandible and at the back of the soft palate before disappearing. They indicate a realignment of muscles attached to the larynx due to the change in pitch, tone focus, and breath control. The patient should be informed that these are excellent signs of progress.

As progress occurs, the patient feels a placement or focus within the mask and is aware that the lower or laryngopharyngeal resonance contributes to the discomfort of speech. The patient begins to maintain the correct pitch and tone focus for longer periods of time. Although the correct voice is used inconsistently, this inconsistency in itself is a sign of progress. The patient becomes able to use the proper tone focus and pitch level with reduced volume so that he can converse in intimate situations in person or on the telephone. The voice lasts longer throughout the day, does not fatigue as easily, and does not cause as much discomfort as it did prior to therapy.

Toward the conclusion of therapy the patient finds that it is effortful or painful to use the old voice or that he is unable to speak in this old voice. The final sign of progress is when the patient no longer needs to concern himself with the process of vocal rehabilitation in order to maintain an efficient or artistic voice.

STAGES OF VOCAL REHABILITATION

Vocal rehabilitation occurs in stages.

1. The patient begins to understand the vocal image, the causes of his voice disorder, and the process of vocal rehabilitation. He is able to produce the correct pitch and tone focus part of the time during the therapy session.

2. The patient is able to produce the correct pitch and tone focus most of the time during the therapy session and is beginning to carry over the new voice to outside situations. He begins to concentrate on breath support in the therapy session. The therapist and patient continue discussions about the vocal role in various situations under different pressures.

3. The patient is able to produce the new voice with coordinated breath support and appropriate volume outside the therapeutic situation automatically. He generally understands and accepts his new voice and new vocal image.

Patients vary in their ability to master these various stages of vocal recovery. Some progress faster in one stage than in another. Patients remaining on plateaus within each stage and regression within a stage or from one stage to another are both normal. Within each stage, there are evidences of progress that can be measured and defined and prognostic signs which determine the outcome of therapy. The therapist must be aware of these stages and the significance of the signs in each stage.

Plateaus

When a patient reaches a plateau, it is necessary to discover the cause, define it, and overcome it. If this phase remains unaltered, the original vocal progress made disappears and the voice disorder may revert to its original strength and disability.

When the patient continues to remain on a plateau, he requires more than understanding and assurance that this phase is normal. Careful definitive vocal analysis is pursued to eliminate this phase. When the patient remains on a plateau for protracted periods of time, it may be helpful if another patient who experienced this difficulty but who has completed therapy is called in to assist the stymied patient.

Regression

Regression or lapses and relapses occur in vocal rehabilitation. Understanding regression, allowing for it, and utilizing it make for knowledgeable, meaningful therapy. The patient should be forewarned about the regression so that he will be able to anticipate the regression and deal with it realistically. For instance, the patient may lose control of the pitch on the phone during an intimate conversation or in a hectic situation. Loss of proper pitch is normal during these conditions. The regression in pitch becomes temporary and brief during the latter stages of pitch control. When the patient attempts to add another variable, such as breath support, to the new voice, he may lose some control of the pitch and the tone focus. The patient always needs assurance that the regression is normal. He is also told that when he realizes he is regressing, he should attempt to recover the correct pitch and tone focus as quickly as possible.

Regression may occur even after therapy is completed. A cold or upper respiratory problem, emotional trauma, neglect of proper vocal habits and/or poor vocal hygiene, physical disability, or intense personality effect can all contribute to the regression.

The pitch and tone focus are the parameters of voice most affected. The pitch may go above or below optimal, or the tone focus leans too heavily upon the lower laryngopharyngeal resonance. Regression is normally short-lived. The patient himself can usually reaffirm his own pitch level and tone focus without the assistance of the voice therapist. If not, a few sessions of vocal therapy will suffice to alert the individual to the condition or circumstance contributing to the regression. A reaffirmation of the correct pitch level and proper tone focus is underscored in therapy, and the patient is once more discharged.

If the former patient is unable to arrange one or two therapy sessions, the therapist may assist him to regain his correct voice by means of a telephone conversation. The therapist can determine incorrect pitch level, tone focus, quality, and rate, detect negative auditory vocal symptoms, and redirect the former patient to his correct voice.

Termination of Therapy

By the time the patient has completed vocal rehabilitation, he should understand the vista of factors that affect his voice and be aware of the answers to surmounting his particular voice problem. Vocal awareness evolves in three phases. In the first phase, the patient realizes that the voice was incorrectly produced *after* speaking. In the second phase, the patient realizes that he is producing his voice incorrectly *during* speaking and attempts to make adjustments and produce the voice correctly. In the third phase, the patient is aware that he is about to use his voice incorrectly *before* speaking. In this last phase, by anticipating the necessary alternatives in the vocal variables, the patient is able to achieve correct vocal production. This indicates the patient is near or ready for discharge.

Some patients are on good vocal behavior during the therapy session; they are using the new voice. Outside of therapy, they report that they revert to the old voice. These patients are not ready for discharge.

The therapist and the patient should agree when therapy should be terminated. The absence of the negative vocal symptoms originally presented, as well as the ease, durability, and automaticity of the new voice, presage the close of therapy. If a growth or lesion was present on the vocal folds initially, the absence of such indicates that vocal rehabilitation is in its closing stage.

The same criteria of voice cannot be used for all patients. Patients who have experienced repeated surgical procedures may not be able to produce an excellent quality of voice. A slightly impaired quality of voice may be acceptable in these patients which would not be acceptable in a patient who has not experienced surgery or who has had perhaps one or two surgical procedures. In the main, however, regardless of the number of surgeries and unless the vocal folds have been irreparably damaged, a good to excellent quality of voice can be achieved.

PROBLEMS OF VOCAL REHABILITATION

The problem with leadership in regard to vocal rehabilitation is more often than not an academic issue. Relationship between the voice therapist and the laryngologist should be a cooperative association. Each has his own role in the vocal rehabilitation process and there should be no conflict as to who is directing the program.

A knowledgeable laryngologist can sometimes assist certain patients with suggestions for vocal improvement. Pleet (1971, personal communication) comments:

> In milder functional misphonias, the qualified otolaryngologist can, in a short time, provide enough information to the patient to significantly alleviate symptoms. These hints consist of providing insight into the functional nature of the disorder, optimal pitch attainment, and avoidance of excessive volume production.

In most dysphonic patients, the laryngologist examines the patient and reports his findings to the voice therapist. The voice therapist, in turn, institutes a program of vocal rehabilitation appropriate to the patient's problem, describing the vocal diagnosis and the program to the laryngologists. Periodic progress reports are afforded the laryngologist. The voice therapist also recommends periodic laryngological examinations when he feels a visual examination will index some progress.

The school speech therapist has special problems. The therapist must have an examination and a report from a laryngologist before working with the child. Since this request must usually go through channels, such as the school nurse to the school doctor to the parent to the laryngologist, very few children are seen for laryngeal examinations. Some parents do not secure a laryngeal examination for their children because of financial difficulties, disinterest, or other personal reasons. Still, other children may be seen by laryngologists who do not feel that voice therapy is relevant.

Another problem is that the speech therapist who is working in the school system may feel inadequately trained to handle voice disorders. Nearly all speech therapists lack voice therapy training that is clinically meaningful. The questions that Froeschels raised in 1948 in his article "Should the Speech Therapist

Be a Voice Therapist?" has been answered in the negative by a number of universities and colleges in the United States. Speech therapists are frustrated by voice cases if they are unprepared clinically by the training institutions to meet with the demands of such cases. Surveys of speech therapists taken at conferences and in classes dealing with vocal rehabilitation reflect the frustrations and disabilities that they have in meeting with voice problems. Many feel inadequate and insecure both in training and in experience with voice disorders. They also report negative vocal symptoms regarding their own speaking voices.

It is ironic to realize that many speech therapists do not have training for their own speaking voices. Speech therapists who have an articulation problem are not readily acceptable as speech therapists. From clinical experience, it has been noted that vocal deficiency or inefficiency is seldom noted in a speech therapist's voice unless it is a marked pitch disorder or quality problem. To become a voice therapist one takes courses and becomes academically certified; he does not need to have his own voice analyzed and developed. Speech therapists may be as guilty of vocal misuse as is the general population. The vocal image and a vocal neurosis also exist among a number of speech therapists.

From contact with speech therapists, it appears that a number are presently unprepared academically and clinically for dealing with voice problems. A recent survey of 403 school speech therapists by means of a questionnaire affords the following information concerning their training, their capabilities with voice patients, and their view of their own vocal efficiency.

How many years have you been a speech therapist?

6.3 average

Highest degree held:

BA	223
MA	150
Ph.D.	2
No Response	28

Certificate of Clinical Competence in Speech:

Yes	246
No	41
No Response	116

Number of courses in the following areas:

	One	Two/more		One	Two/more
Voice science	182	18	Psychology of voice ..	52	9
Advanced v.s.	140	3	Principles of voice		
Exper. phonetics	111	8	training	55	11
Anatomy	136	40	Voice disorders	155	21
Physiology	124	25	Others (Neurology)	15	1

Please list the number of voice cases you have worked with in each of the following categories:

	Adults	Children
Functional dysphonia (no growths)	72	561
Falsetto	15	126
Nodules or nodes	39	470
Polyps	36	53
Contact ulcer	20	14
Paralyzed vocal fold	17	46
Spastic dysphonia	5	36
Hysterical aphonia	18	24
Bowed vocal folds		2
Other	35	81

54 therapists have seen adults
92 therapists have seen children
‾‾
146

Of these 146, 44 therapists have seen both adults and children; therefore, only 128 therapists have worked with voice cases.

(Author's note: From the answers on the above question, it would appear that some therapists are somewhat confused in their diagnosis of childhood dysphonias, i.e. paralyzed vocal fold, spastic dysphonia, hysterical aphonia.)

Are you unable to work with voice cases for any of the following reasons?

Speech problems are given priority	109
Voice cases not referred	147
Difficulty in obtaining a laryngological examination	208
Difficulty in educating the parent that the child has a voice problem	147
Other	35
No Response	86

Do you feel competent in voice therapy with adults?

Yes	44
No	264
No Response	95

Do you feel competent in voice therapy with children?

Yes 76
No 246
No Response 81

If you feel competent, which of the following applies?

Excellent coursework in voice 42
Good training in vocal rehabilitation 50
Training of your own voice in speech pathology course 30
Training of your own voice outside the school curriculum ... 32
Improvement in voice cases 61
Voice cases remained resolved 36

If you feel incompetent, which of the following applies?

Little or no coursework in voice 133
Little or no supervision in vocal rehabilitation 222
Little or inadequate training of your own voice 98
Little or no improvement in voice cases 69
Improvement followed by relapse in voice cases 31
Not enough voice cases seen 216

Do you avoid taking voice cases because you feel inadequately trained or incompetent to handle the symptoms?

Yes 180
No 161
No Response 62

Would you want more or less training for your own speaking voice?

More 279
Less 20
No Response 104

Please specify the extent of voice training you received for your own voice during speech pathology courses and/or other academic training:

Hours	Therapists	Hours	Therapists
2	12	12	3
3	47	15	1
4	12	16	2
5	8	17	1
6	17	18	2
8	10	20	3
9	7	24	1
10	2	25	1
11	1	50	1

52	1	200	1
58	1	300	1
70	1		
100	1		137

What is your evaluation of the training?

Excellent	20	Poor	19
Good	38	No response	16
Fair	44		

Have you experienced any of these symptoms during or after speaking?

Tired voice	113
Neck aches or pains	26
Pressure at sternum	6
Neck muscle cording	10
Lump in throat	45
Tickling, tearing, or burning sensation in throat	57
Throat clearing	106
Coughing	49
Repeated sore throats	29
Voice breaks and skips	34
Loss of voice	33

Almost twenty-five years ago Williamson in 1946 investigated the adequacy of voice training. He (p. 145) states:

> For two decades I had found it more difficult to engage a teacher equipped to train the speaking voice and to remedy voice defects than to find almost any other kind of speech teacher. An instructor with an advanced degree from any one of our graduate speech departments can usually be counted upon to teach the greater number of subjects in our field—occasionally including the correction of major speech defects—but not to deal adequately with the voice.

Williamson (p. 146) quotes from a letter written by Dr. Robert West, who expresses his view:

> There are very few persons in the field of speech who know enough about voice to treat its disorders. I quite agree with you that the field of voice therapy is one of the weakest links in the armor of most of our clinicians.

Williamson (p. 160) summarizes:

> It may be said in general conclusion that the authorities . . . express uniform dissatisfaction with our present training of voice therapists, and a number of them advance definite, well-outlined pro-

posals for the improvement of scientific knowledge of voice, of the use of scientific instruments, and of clinical methods. Though pointing to a like need for improvement of instruction in the craft of voice training, they suggest, however, no similarly well-thought-out plan for remedying the weaknesses of this important phase of our training.

Brodnitz (1966b, p. 270) affirms the problem of clinical training in voice: "Those of us who are engaged in teaching, however, have been aware for quite some time that voice is still a stepchild of the training programs in speech pathology." He (p. 270) further writes: "It is a common complaint among the younger clinicians that they feel inadequate when confronted with a voice patient because their training has not given them sufficient knowledge of the disorders of voice." He (p. 272) continues:

> The number of programs, however, which do not include systematic training in the handling of patients with disorders of voice is uncomfortably high. Too many do not teach disorders of voice at all or deal with them as a minor subject, lack the technical facilities for teaching this subject, have neither sufficient numbers of voice patients nor systematic collections of voice recordings, and do not get the benefit of interdisciplinary teamwork.

In the intervening period of nineteen years between Williamson and Brodnitz, the situation does not seem to have improved.

Darley (1969) discusses the importance of clinical activity and the need for better trained clinicians in all areas. He (p. 146) writes: "I believe our students are not being inspired with a vision of the opportunities, the rewards, and the worth of clinical endeavors." He (p. 147) continues:

> But I get the impression that our teachers are afraid to bare their skills or the lack of them to their students. They talk about the kinds of things one should do but they are unwilling to demonstrate them.
>
> . . . .
>
> There are people abroad in the land who are doing clinical work every day. Somehow in our training programs we must exploit their skills either by offering them enough money and equal opportunities for promotion to lure them into the educational institutions or by getting our students out into some kind of off-campus practicum experience in the settings where these people are working. . . .
>
> Further, the clinical supervision provided should be more than

nominal. The supervisor cannot find out what the clinician is doing right or wrong by reading logs written by him last week. . . . The supervisor must be there—often—and critique—regularly.

In summary, Darley (p. 148) states: "The honest clinician is the person least likely to suggest a dichotomy between good patient care and good research. They are inextricably intertwined in his daily work."

Another major problem is the dichotomy between the research and the clinical activities in the field of voice. Unfortunately, from clinical observation, some researchers who study the functions of the vocal mechanism do not do clinical work and many clinicians in vocal therapy do not do research. Too often research is done with no application being made to assist the clinician with the clinical aspect of the voice problem.

Powers (1955) clearly and succinctly points out this dichotomy and other problems which exist, including the prevalent use of graduate students as subjects in studies and the scientific jargon utilized in research reports. Regarding research activities, she (p. 6) comments: "Each is too limited in scope, deals with too few cases or cases not comparable with those in other studies, deals with too narrow a range of behavior or with too limited a method of measurement to add importantly to our knowledge." She (p. 6) continues:

Another explanation of the present divisive trend lies in the fact that most of our research is centered in our universities, whereas most of the therapy goes on outside the universities, particularly in our public school programs.

This author agrees with Powers that too many clinical reports in the field of vocal rehabilitation involve the reporting of a limited number of cases. Not only should the laboratory research be related in a practical manner to clinical therapy but also reports of clinical activities should include meaningful numbers of subjects or patients.

GENERAL REASONS FOR FAILURES IN VOCAL REHABILITATION

There are many reasons for failure in vocal rehabilitation. Extreme resistance to the concept of vocal rehabilitation exists in many patients in and of itself. The voice patient has seldom, if ever, heard of vocal rehabilitation. Also, because of the lack of education relevant to the speaking voice and its apparatus, the voice patient often has a bedrock of vocal mythology, which leads to the rejection of therapy.

The voice patient may be of the view that he is alone and abnormal in experiencing a voice problem. More often than not he may be prone to seek a panacea or an exercise or two which will remove his voice disorder overnight. He is quite unable to grasp the fact that vocal misuse has created his vocal symptoms and that vocal rehabilitation will remove these symptoms. Only with time, vocal improvement, and resolution of the negative vocal symptoms does the patient begin to assign cause and effect, i.e. wrong pitch, incorrect tone focus, emotional and psychological tensions and vocal images to the voice disorder.

Patients are usually referred to a voice therapist only after hoarseness is recurrent and only after the voice problem has prevailed for a number of years. This referral is usually made after palliative measures have been attempted but have not been curative or substantive. By this time, the speaking voice is seriously impaired and is possibly creating emotional trauma. These patients require a great deal of time and effort to rehabilitate.

Ironically, there are those who do not want a good voice, who do not need a good voice, or who do not care about producing a good voice. These individuals are not interested in vocal rehabilitation.

A patient may not be initially committed to a program of vocal rehabilitation. Even though he begins therapy, this individual stands little chance of being rehabilitated until (1) the extent of the disability and the degree of discomfort adversely affect the patient; and (2) the communicative impairment and the aesthetic vocal devastation cause sufficient negative comments and reactions from those who are important or meaningful to the individual.

Some individuals are uninterested in vocal rehabilitation because they either do not understand it and/or do not believe in it. Of those who have had surgery, some may believe that the growth will not return. Others decide they will take a chance on its not returning. If it does return, they will undergo another surgery. They feel this is easier, more meaningful, or less both-ersome to them than changing their voice through vocal rehabil-itation.

Patients who have undergone surgery frequently anticipate a return of the clear pregrowth voice following surgery. If the voice does not return, vocal rehabilitation may be necessary. Some patients are unable to accept the need for vocal rehabilita-tion or abide with a program of vocal rehabilitation following a surgical procedure. Brodnitz (1963, p. 152) explains:

> The concept of vocal rehabilitation is not easily grasped by the pa-tient. He expects the surgeon to free him from an impairment of his voice and cannot understand why he has to submit to a somewhat lengthy period of vocal training after successful surgery.

Some patients express the desire to alter old vocal patterns and acquire a new voice, but they are unwilling to practice and cooperate with the voice therapist. Their attitude is that thera-py must be done for them, not by them. Others are unable to take the time, the effort, the self-responsibility, and the vocal concentration to establish a new vocal identity. Other patients believe that by merely attending the therapy session with some token effort for vocal carry-over the voice problem will be quick-ly resolved. Token support results in failure.

The circumstances under which a few voice patients begin or continue vocal rehabilitation preclude complete and even partial vocal recovery. A few patients seek financial settlements for loss or impairment of the speaking voice through accidents. They are prone to vocal failure by denying vocal practice, although they may well have vocal insight and understanding of the voice disorder involved.

Some patients drop out of therapy because they do not obtain immediate relief or resolution of the voice problem, although they have been forewarned the process will take time and effort.

"Traveling" voice patients usually are not successful. These patients move from one therapist to another, faulting each and denying any the ability or knowledgeability to assist them. They seldom listen to instructions or follow directions. They are too busy concocting reasons and rationales for finding whatever therapy they are given unsatisfactory and dissatisfying. The therapist should suspect that he may be seeing a "traveling" voice patient when the patient mentions that he has worked with two or more therapists without achieving any results.

Patients may discontinue therapy because of economic reasons. Some patients may not be able to afford therapy. Others do not wish to pay a fee for training the speaking voice; they are not convinced of the importance or relevance of vocal rehabilitation.

A not inconsequential factor in the cessation of vocal therapy is the denial of payment by insurance companies. Recompense for vocal rehabilitation in private therapy or in clinics is highly variable. Vocal rehabilitation is a relatively unknown area to insurance companies. A number of companies exclude vocal rehabilitation by nonmention of it in the list of services that are covered by insurance rather than by specific exclusion.

Some patients are in town only briefly for surgery and/or vocal rehabilitation. The length of time may not be sufficient for a complete recovery even though intensive therapy is utilized. Needed follow-up sessions are impossible with these patients.

Strange as it may seem, patients who make good vocal progress too quickly may drop out of therapy before they are ready for discharge. An amelioration in the quality of voice from husky or hoarse to clear and a decrease in the negative vocal symptoms may influence the patient to terminate therapy. He presumes either that he is now able to handle his own problem or that his voice disorder is over. Relapse in these cases is to be expected.

Children experience failure in vocal rehabilitation for similar reasons. They may not understand the purpose of therapy; they may not wish to practice; they may not want to change their voices. Children receiving therapy in the school system may not want to miss certain classes or they may not want to be singled out as "different" for attending speech class. Parents may not want their children in vocal rehabilitation for many of the same reasons patients do not want therapy.

Failure in vocal rehabilitation for both adults and children is a many-faceted phenomenon. It occurs for many reasons under various circumstances. What creates failure in one patient may well create success in another. Fortunately, failure is not as prevalent in vocal rehabilitation as is success.

PSYCHOLOGICAL REASONS FOR FAILURE IN VOCAL REHABILITATION

One of the main reasons for failure in vocal rehabilitation is the patient's inability to reject the old vocal image and to accept the new vocal image. The old vocal image may have become the role identity. If so, the patient may be unable to mentally or physically give up this vocal role despite intellectual realization that the old voice or old vocal image is inappropriate for him. He may prefer to remain vocally crippled.

To change the misuse and abuse of voice to proper vocal usage requires a new vocal image. The new vocal image is one of the most devastating attributes in all of vocal rehabilitation. The patient almost always reacts sharply and markedly against it. Regardless of the verbal willingness to overcome the voice disorder, the new vocal image is simply too much for some patients, and so they discontinue therapy. Identification of the vocal image and the reasons for it too early in therapy may be too threatening for one patient while another needs this knowledge early in order to overcome his problem and achieve success. If the new vocal image is introduced slowly, the patient may drop because therapy is not progressing fast enough. Failure will almost always occur if the patient is unable to resolve the vocal identity crisis. The therapist must guide the patient through this crucial period of therapy.

Some voice patients will fail to regain a natural or efficient voice because they do not want such a voice. They are pleased with the voice they present though it is basically hoarse and misused. Individuals associated with or related to the patient may appreciate the pathological voice, and the patient is willing to accept the views of those who like the hoarse or misused voice. The patient himself may like the pathological voice and want to continue it.

There are other patients who continue a voice disorder because it satisfies their internal drives and needs. They want to express and exploit a vocal disability and vocal failure as proof of internal problems. To these patients, the disturbed voice is an outward manifestation of the internal disorder, stamping them as being troubled or emotionally complicated individuals. In essence, the vocal disability satisfies a neurotic need and is sufficiently fulfilling to warrant its continuance.

Some voice patients fear recovery of their voices because it means they will have to engage in a situation which they wish to evade or confront a person whom they are unwilling or unable to encounter. Lack of voice or impairment of the voice may help them avoid confrontations, involvements, or expression of feelings, and thereby allows them to circumvent threatening people or situations.

Vocal rehabilitation failure also ensues because the patient does not wish to allow the therapist to be successful. The patient pursues methods which will insure failure because he does not want the therapist to consider him a resolved case.

Vocal psychotherapy may be inadequate for patients who present some of these psychological reasons for failure in vocal rehabilitation. The patient who courts vocal failure may have serious emotional problems which should be resolved. Psychotherapy may be necessary prior to or in conjunction with vocal rehabilitation for these patients.

THE THERAPIST AND FAILURE IN VOCAL REHABILITATION

The ineptness of the therapist is a consideration which seldom is mentioned in the literature. The therapist may be an excellent speech therapist, but he may not be adequately trained in vocal rehabilitation as previously discussed. The therapist may be mechanistically able to train a voice but is unable to work with the personality aspect or vocal psychotherapy. Inept vocal therapy contributes to vocal disorders.

Failure involves inappropriate words, thoughts, directions, attitudes, and reactions in general, as well as inappropriate steps in vocal rehabilitation. The therapist may fail in not doing or in not giving something at the right time to the right patient. He may also fail in not determining the reasons a patient is failing, reasons that under careful and full investigation might afford a different approach in therapy.

The therapist's rigidity in adhering to a given vocal rehabilitation regimen which meets with his needs and fulfillment but not those of the patient may create failure. For example, some patients are unwilling to work at mechanical exercises and prefer to chat in order to learn a new pitch and new correct voice. The therapist must adapt the therapy to the patient. Some patients need to progress rapidly and others need to move slowly. The therapist must pace the therapy to the patient's ability and understanding.

Personality structure being variable, it is impossible for a voice therapist to work successfully with all patients for a resolution of their vocal problems. It is not realistic to expect the therapist to be all things to all patients. The therapist may not be able to experience rapport with, nor empathy for, nor relate to, a patient. The patient may experience the same lack of interest, concern, and authenticity with the therapist. The therapist can minimize the differences in temperament between himself and the patient often but not always. Such is also true of the patient.

Failure in vocal rehabilitation is necessary and vital to make the therapist realize his fullest potential. It also forces him to review himself and his therapy sufficiently, so that he learns to reduce the number of failures. The therapist who understands the various reasons for failure, whether due to the therapist or to the patient, has a more realistic review of vocal rehabilitation. He, therefore, can assess his abilities and disabilities with insight in a more meaningful context. He learns to be a more knowledgeable and competent therapist as well as a more humane and empathetic human being. Failure is a spur to eventual fulfillment of the potential of the therapist as a therapist and as a self-sufficient human being.

PART 4

VOCAL REHABILITATION: THERAPY FOR FUNCTIONAL AND ORGANIC DYSPHONIAS

The therapy techniques which have been described are applicable, with adjustments and adaptations, to most types of functional and organic dysphonias. Because different age groups present unique problems, specific consideration is given to these groups in this section. The most commonly seen dysphonias are also discussed with further suggestions for therapy. Some, such as spastic dysphonia and esophageal voice, which have not been analyzed previously in this book are outlined in more detail.

At the end of this section, charts are presented listing the number of patients seen who had experienced each dysphonia, the age range, the sex, the length of therapy, and the result of therapy. At the close of the discussion of each dysphonia, summary statements derived from the charts are provided. The author suggests a brief perusal of the discussion entitled "Results" in the last section of the book for a complete understanding of the terminology used in the charts and in the summaries.

DYSPHONIAS BY AGE GROUPINGS

Childhood Dysphonias

The incidence of voice disorders in children has been estimated to be 5 percent by Frick (1960) and 6 percent by Senturia and Wilson (1968). Hoarseness occurs in 7.1 percent according to Baynes (1966). Curry (1949), investigating males, estimated 55 percent were hoarse—husky at ten years of age and 80 percent hoarse—husky at fourteen years of age. Lore (1950, p. 825) finds: "Hoarseness in children is far more widespread than is usually supposed." Froeschels (1943, p. 130) reports: "Many children, especially school children, show symptoms of hyperfunction, and a smaller number exhibit symptoms of hypofunction." Negative vocal symptoms are the same for children as for adults (Cooper, 1970e, 1971b).

Most voice disorders in children are functional, the most common type being functional misphonia. Some children have been known to experience hysterical aphonia and spastic dysphonia; falsetto may be found in adolescents. Children may have organic dysphonias. The most frequent type noted is nodules, followed by polyps. Papillomatosis occurs infrequently. Contact ulcer is rarely seen.

Vocal misuse and abuse are the most common causes of most childhood dysphonias (Cooper, 1971b). Murphy (1967) writes that the so-called Singer's nodule is basically caused by vocal abuse. Moses (1940) attributes the impairments of children's voices to choral singing in schools. Froeschels (1943) cites poor reading, speaking, and singing as causes of hoarseness and hyperfunction. Pahn (1966) finds that malfunctions of the speaking and singing voice in childhood leads to malfunctions of the voice in adults.

Variable combinations of vocal misuse and vocal abuse, in this author's experience, have begun or continued a childhood dysphonia. In many preschool children the optimal pitch of voice as well as a balanced tone focus in the oronasopharynx is apparently inherent and often may be clinically noted. Factors which negatively affect the voice apparently occur after this age. These factors may be vocal abuse due to excessive shouting and/or vocal misuse due to singing in the wrong range, development of a vocal image that involves the imitation of an inappropriate pitch level and tone focus, illnesses which may cause protracted body fatigue, upper respiratory infection or cold which may result in a lowered pitch level, imitation of a poor vocal model (teacher as well as parent; no vocal image involved), inept suggestions from teachers ("Speak up to reach the back of the room," which causes the child to shout instead of projecting), lack of vocal knowledge or vocal training (child is not taught to project voice or to refrain from poor vocal hygiene), and imitation of an inappropriate voice for the child (no vocal image involved). Emotional problems can also contribute to the onset and continuation of a voice disorder.

Voice reeducation for children is outlined by Wilson (1962a). Vocal rehabilitation techniques adapted from adults to children are not meaningful, according to O'Neil and McGee (1962). From clinical experience this would depend upon the individual child and what type of therapy is being done for an adult.

This author has found that direct vocal rehabilitation with some modification works well with children. The child is given the correct pitch and proper tone focus. Therapy techniques which may be used with children are as follows:

1. Play therapy in which the child verbalizes while playing. The therapist uses direct vocal rehabilitation in guiding the child to the correct pitch and tone focus.

2. Role therapy in which the child becomes voice conscious and assumes different voices as he tells stories or acts out plays.

3. Practice with a tape recorder or Language Master. The therapist specifies the correct and incorrect pitch levels and tone focuses as the child practices and listens to his own voice.

4. Counseling of parent(s) and/or sibling(s). The voice problem is discussed and ways of helping at home are suggested. Examples are reminding the patient, at appropriate times, to use the correct voice, praise for using this voice, and direct practice at home with the parent.

5. Teaching the child projection. The child must be shown how to project the voice instead of shouting, since most children have the need to express themselves loudly at times.

The child requires understanding of his vocal demands and vocal needs by both therapist and parent(s). The therapist must afford the child the means to meet those vocal demands in the new voice. The parent(s) must support the therapist in his demands of the child. For the child, vocal rehabilitation must be pleasurable, interesting, and activating of participation by the child.

The child must be able to express any feelings or thoughts in therapy without penalty. Nemec (1961) finds that hyperkinetic dysphonia reveals aggressive behavior. Therefore, he feels that hyperkinetic dysphonia in children requires psychotherapy. Our experience has also revealed that vocal psychotherapy is necessary. The child frequently has a vocal image, and the older the child, the stronger the vocal image. The attraction or rejection of voice types must be explored. Vocal culture and vocal neurosis influence young children as well as adults. Mosby (1970, p. 891), in discussing one case, concludes:

> In summary, then, this case study suggests psychotherapy should be considered as treatment for cases of functional voice deviations which are resistive to the usual voice therapy procedures. When used in conjunction with the practice of making specific vocal changes, psychotherapy may facilitate improvement and reinforce the client in maintaining such gains.*

Intensive vocal therapy is usually not necessary. The child should be seen thirty to forty-five minutes per session, once or twice weekly.

Good vocal hygiene must be instituted, as follows:

1. Restriction of activities which involve shouting if the child is unable to refrain from shouting. The parent must intervene and remove the child from these situations.

2. Termination of choral singing. The child may be singing in the wrong pitch level or singing too loudly.

---

* Reprinted with permission of author and publisher. D. P. Mosby, Psychotherapy versus voice therapy for a child with a deviant voice, a case study. *Perceptual and Motor Skills*, 1970, 30:887-891.

Unfortunately, children are seldom referred for vocal rehabilitation, since hoarseness seems to be accepted as normal in children. Physicians often advise waiting to see if the problem will abate at puberty. Many children who do enter vocal rehabilitation have a favorable prognosis, provided that there is parental cooperation for the younger child and interest and concern for his own dysphonia by the older child.

Adolescent Dysphonias

In the adolescent, functional dysphonia involves mainly functional misphonia and falsetto. Spastic dysphonia and hysterical aphonia occur rarely. The main organic type is nodules.

According to Moses (1940, p. 446): "Many voice disturbances in all stages of life are results of mutation, or change, of voice." Clinical experience with males would tend partially to support this position. When the male experiences the change of voice at puberty, the voice may drop to the basal or near basal pitch level and remains at that level. Continued use of this voice creates dysphonias.

Negative vocal symptoms are usually as severe, as frequent, and as extensive in the adolescent patient as in the adult patient. The falsetto voice especially presents noticeable negative auditory vocal symptoms. Because of the relatively frequent occurrence of the falsetto voice in the adolescent and because of its specialized therapy, a full discussion is presented under "Falsetto."

Vocal rehabilitation with the adolescent voice patient is extremely challenging. The major problem in therapy with this age category is the lack of motivation. The therapist must find various ways to activate the adolescent to concern himself with his voice. Good vocal hygiene may not be recognized to be of essential significance to these patients. Muma, Laeder, and Webb (1968, p. 581) conclude:

> It was apparent that persons with obviously different voice qualities do not differ appreciably in peer evaluation from persons with normal voice quality. . . . According to these findings, speech pathologists need not expect to find personal and social implications of voice quality aberrations of adolescents.

Associate therapy may not be apropos with this age group. The parent(s) should be aware of the purpose and techniques of vocal rehabilitation as well as the problems involved, but a parent does not usually become an active, integral participant in the rehabilitative process.

Vocal rehabilitation techniques for the adolescent are similar to those for the adult. As always, the therapy must be adapted to the individual patient. Some other therapy techniques for the adolescent are outlined in Wilson (1962b). Vocal rehabilitation with adolescents has been generally successful.

Geriatric Dysphonias

In dysphonias which involve geriatric patients, the organic types include growths or lesions on the vocal folds as well as neurological involvements, such as paralytic dysphonia and Parkinson's disease. Geriatric patients have experienced routine and long-term misuse and abuse of the speaking voice which eventuates into classical negative vocal symptoms and dysphonias. The aging process alone affects the voice more in some patients than in others and in different ways in different patients. Generally, the aging process of the laryngeal mechanism need not affect the durability and comfort of the speaking voice.

The geriatric patient seems to be more readily responsive to physical fatigue, poor health, illness, and mental affective reactions, such as depression, which reflect themselves in a lowered pitch of voice and in a tone focus in the laryngopharynx. The volume is usually reduced. The quality of voice is usually either hoarse or breathy. Upper chest breathing prevails for speech. Although the process of vocal rehabilitation for the geriatric patient is similar to the routine previously discussed, more extended vocal psychotherapy may be necessary. Although most geriatric patients are not actively seeking a vocal image, they retain the misused voice which has become a firmly established vocal pattern from the influence of an earlier vocal image. The geriatric patient often needs a new vocal identity, so the new voice is accepted and used by the patient.

McGlone and Hollien (1963, p. 170) report "that speaking pitch level of women probably varies little throughout adult life. . . ." Mysak (1959) finds that in elderly adult males the average fundamental pitch level rises with progressive aging. From clinical experience, nearly all of the geriatric patients seen, both males and females, have been using a habitual pitch level which was below the optimal pitch level; however, most geriatric patients seen were between sixty and seventy years of age.

These patients are seldom referred for vocal rehabilitation. Physicians may be unaware of the vocal misuse in functional and organic dysphonias or unaware of vocal rehabilitation. Other physicians may feel that vocal rehabilitation is not relevant for these patients.

Geriatric patients themselves may be unreceptive to vocal rehabilitation. The reasons for this are lack of strong physician support for the program, lack of understanding and/or belief in vocal retraining, and lack of motivation to change the voice. These patients seldom realize that their voices are misused.

Geriatric patients can be helped by vocal rehabilitation in many cases. For vocal rehabilitation to be successful, there must be a strong physician referral, cooperation between the physician and the voice therapist (Cooper, 1970g), family support and motivation.

FUNCTIONAL MISPHONIA

Therapy for patients with functional misphonia has been previously described. See Charts 1 and 2 for these patients with the number and percentages.

From Charts 1 and 2, the following conclusions may be drawn:

1. Of the 486 patients seen, 341 or 70.2 percent entered therapy.

2. Of the 341 patients entering therapy, 313 or 91.8 percent completed therapy.

3. Of the 313 patients completing therapy, 51 or 16.3 percent had long-term therapy and 262 or 83.7 percent had short-term therapy.

4. Of the 313 patients completing therapy, the results were excellent, 233 or 74.4 percent; good, 53 or 16.9 percent; fair, 27 or 8.6 percent.

5. The comparison between males and females seen: males, 244 or 50.2 percent; females, 242 or 49.8 percent.

FALSETTO

The falsetto voice has a specific sound which distinguishes it from all other types of voices. It is extremely high-pitched, representing the uppermost pitch range of the entire speaking voice. Other auditory symptoms include a thin quality, a wavering tone, a restricted pitch range, a monotonous pitch, and a lack of volume usually. This voice develops in the male during or following puberty. Four female patients with falsetto voice were seen by this author. Lerman and Duffy (1970, p. 26) did research

> . . . to determine if falsetto voice quality could be distinguished from normal high pitch on the basis of perception of voice quality. . . . Judges identified the source of phonation as "falsetto," "normal," "female," or "child." The results indicate that: (1) Seventy percent of the falsetto tones were perceived correctly by the listeners. (2) The normal male high pitch had the lowest percentage of correct identification, and was most often misidentified as male falsetto. (3) Female vocal production was correctly identified 66 percent of the time. It had a much higher misidentification with children's voice than with the other two vocal samples. (4) Children's production were the most accurately perceived (94 percent).

Two main points of view exist regarding the etiology of the falsetto voice (Satou and Cooper, 1968). One viewpoint posits that the falsetto voice is utilized because the individual does not know how to use his voice; the solution is one of vocal reeducation. The other view is that the etiology is due to psychological factors, i.e. inner emotional conflicts, such as identification problems, unresolved maternal difficulties, and a wish to remain infantile or childish; the solution is psychiatric treatment or psychotherapy. Thus, the falsetto voice may be created and continued because of lack of vocal training or because of emotional and psychological needs of the individual to continue a given status, position, role, and vocal identity which may afford the individual stability and security.

From clinical experience, it would be reasonable to report that approximately 50 percent of all falsetto voices fall within the realm of the emotional and psychological as actuating and continuing factors. Approximately 50 percent of all falsetto patients yield reasonably well to direct vocal rehabilitation. The length of therapy is usually from three to six months.

Vocal psychotherapy is an inherent aspect of direct vocal rehabilitation. The change from a falsetto voice to a baritone or bass voice requires a variable degree of vocal psychotherapy depending upon the ego strength of the patient, external pressures and circumstances about him, and his needs and demands. If the therapist is unable to provide vocal psychotherapy or psychotherapy as needed, the therapist may seek a combined program of treatment for the patient utilizing the services of a psychologist or psychiatrist for the psychotherapy.

Associate therapy in vocal rehabilitation for falsetto voice may be used selectively. Even when direct vocal rehabilitation is successful and brief vocal psychotherapy is sufficient, it has been found that the patient's family may object to the new voice and is negative to its mastery in some cases. The resolution of the falsetto voice requires sufficient character and personality strength to maintain a new vocal image and vocal identity.

The individual who has a falsetto voice may be directed to the basal or near basal pitch level initially. It has been found that the abrupt pitch change to the basal pitch level is much more successful than lowering the pitch to the optimal pitch level for several reasons. The patient usually has a tendency to revert to his old pitch level. By using a lowered or lowest pitch there is sufficient contrast so that the patient is better able to monitor himself and is more aware when he reverts to the old falsetto voice. The optimal pitch level also may not give the patient a stable reference point; the basal pitch gives a definite reference point since the individual simply drops as low as he can. If the new pitch level is very low, it enables the patient to get a totally new sound, vocal identity, and muscular realignment.

Psychologically, the patient may not accept the new pitch level, but he is reassured that this new pitch level is only temporary, and that it will hasten the development of a new and better voice. Once he masters this new low pitch, the pitch is raised to the optimal pitch level. The patient then more readily accepts the optimal pitch level as being less threatening to himself and to others than was the basal pitch level. van Thal (1967) also initially forces the patient's pitch level to the bottom of the pitch range and it is raised later in therapy.

If the patient is able to hear the optimal pitch level and maintain it, there is no need to force the pitch level down to the basal pitch level. The approach of lowering the pitch level to the basal is used for those patients who cannot monitor the optimal pitch level easily and quickly. If the patient cannot identify this pitch level after a few sessions, the therapist may find it feasible to utilize a lowered pitch level by the patient for contrast, identification, and ear training.

It is interesting to note that whether the patient drops the pitch level to the basal pitch or to the optimal pitch he experiences negative vocal reactions, hearing himself as forced, hoarse, superficial, and artificial. The falsetto patient has the same reaction to his new vocal identity, if not more so, than does the individual who has to have his pitch raised.

Exercises to lower the falsetto voice are as follows:

1. The vowels /o/ and /u/ are the initial sounds used to change the falsetto voice to a normal voice. The patient is directed to say /o/ repeatedly at the lowest comfortable pitch level until he can master the production of this vowel in isolation. The /o/ is recorded on a Language Master card and replayed after each trial, with the therapist counseling the patient as to the acceptability or nonacceptability of the sound. Within a few sessions, the patient is able to monitor himself and afford himself correct kinesthetic and auditory cues that identify the correct pitch level. In the beginning, this practice is usually done on a pitch level which is below the optimal pitch level.

2. When the patient is able to produce the /o/ at the lowest pitch level, the therapist may decide to proceed to the vowel /u/ followed by /a/, or /i/, so that each of the vowels in succession are basically produced, monitored, and mastered. Another approach is to move from the vowel /o/ to a vowel and number combination "/o/-one, /o/-two" to ten and then a vowel, number, and phrase combination, followed by vowel, number, and sentence

combination. Additional approaches may be to combine two vowels with a number, such as "/o/-/u/-one, /o/-/u/-two" (to ten), followed by two vowels, a number, and a phrase, and finally, the use of two vowels, a number, and a sentence. The words, phrases and sentences are from word and sentence lists.

3. Whatever approach with the vowels and numbers is taken, recording and replaying on the Language Master cards is ever constant, with the therapist guiding the patient as to the correct sound. The therapist must determine what variations or approaches are best for each individual patient. Spontaneous speech is next utilized, using a single vowel, such as an /o/, or two vowels, such as /o/-/u/ or a vowel and a number combination, "/o/-one" or "/o/-/u/-one" followed by a spontaneous sentence. An example would be "/o/-one, I am feeling very well today."

4. When spontaneous speech has been mastered at this lowered or basal pitch level, the patient's pitch is brought up to the optimal level. It is simple enough to force the patient's pitch down to the near basal or basal pitch level, but the therapist must not allow the patient to remain at this pitch level or else a future dysphonia is in the making. A basal or near basal pitch level will create pharyngeal and/or laryngeal tensions with subsequent vocal impairment.

If the patient is unable to produce a vowel sound at the low pitch, other methods are available. Forceful vocalization at the lowest possible pitch, using any vowel, with possible use of pressure upon the midsection as the patient lies supine, sits in a chair, or stands. Another useful method is to lower the pitch one tone at a time, slowly acclimatizing the patient to a lower pitch. Another technique is to have the patient turn his head to the side and cough. He then utters a vowel at the level of the cough which may well reflect the true pitch of the patient. The spontaneous natural laugh is often an index to the optimal pitch level and natural voice of the patient with a falsetto voice. The new voice for the falsetto voice patient is nearly always baritone or bass, with essentially good if not outstanding vocal quality.

Individuals who change from a falsetto to a normal voice

must expect to experience new and additional laryngeal and pharyngeal symptoms for a temporary period of time. With the mastery of the new voice, sensory, auditory, and visual symptoms of the falsetto voice should disappear.

Some individuals with a falsetto voice are desirous of gradually changing from the falsetto to a natural voice. This is done by introducing the normal voice in selected situations with specific individuals, progressively widening the number of situations and types of people with whom the natural voice is used. A number of individuals with falsetto voice are well aware that they have two voices: the falsetto voice and the natural voice, which is usually referred to as the "other" voice by falsetto patients. They are either unable to maintain the other voice or are fearful of utilizing the other voice. Therefore, the programmed exercises afford them control of the new voice and the vocal psychotherapy or psychotherapy affords them emotional or psychological support for the use of the new voice.

The falsetto voice demands a keen appreciation of the emotional and psychological influences on the patient by the therapist. This understanding in combination with a mechanical therapeutic means of programmed exercises develops the normal speaking voice. Bryngelson (1954) describes a therapy program for the falsetto voice.

A review of our cases over the last ten years reveals a breakdown by numbers and percentages in Charts 3 and 4.

From Charts 3 and 4, the following conclusions may be drawn:

1. Of the 34 patients seen, 22 or 64.7 percent entered therapy.

2. Of the 22 patients entering therapy, 20 or 90.9 percent completed therapy.

3. Of the 20 patients completing therapy, 5 or 25 percent had long-term therapy and 15 or 75 percent had short-term therapy.

4. Of the 20 patients completing therapy, the results were excellent, 15 or 75 percent; good, 2 or 10 percent; fair, 3 or 15 percent.

5. The comparison between males and females seen: males, 30 or 88.2 percent; females, 4 or 11.8 percent.

VENTRICULAR PHONATION

The diagnosis of ventricular phonation is often made by the laryngologist as the result of a laryngeal examination. Jackson and Jackson (1935b) find that 4 percent of all patients with hoarse voices examined by them were utilizing ventricular phonation. From clinical experience, ventricular phonation is a rather rare condition and from a review of cases seen is equivalent to less than 1 percent. Descriptions and discussions of ventricular phonation have been made by Voelker (1935, 1942), Van Riper and Irwin (1958), Arnold and Pinto (1960), Freud (1962), and others. Ventricular phonation is often confused with hoarseness or the vocal fry. Ventricular phonation has a specific and distinct sound to it because it utilizes vibration of the false vocal folds and because these folds are lacking in flexibility. Generally, the pitch is extremely low, the quality is markedly hoarse, and the volume is quite limited which affords the voice little carrying power. True ventricular phonation does not easily yield to vocal rehabilitation.

Ventricular phonation may be self-induced and caused by vocal misuse, especially too low a pitch level, and inept tone focus with too much emphasis on laryngopharyngeal resonance. The etiology of ventricular phonation may be attributed to a vocal image that prompts the individual to speak in as low a pitch as possible. This type of voice may start with a cold. The individual pampers the voice since the throat may be irritated or the vocal folds inflamed. He is under the misguided impression that reduced volume and lowered pitch during a cold will conserve the voice. He may like this low pitch and continue it after the cold has abated. Harris (1960, p. 183) concurs:

> Most of these people who have so called dysphonia plica ventricularis are very proud of their lower pitched voices and would not change if they could. I think they could. I think that in many instances they find during some acute inflammation that this lower pitched voice is more likable and they learn how to produce it, just as one learns how to speak with the false cords after operation, such as laryngo-fissure.

Freud (1962, p. 340) finds: "This kind of voice is symptomatic for an insecure, anxious or even neurotic personality." Fred

(1962) mentions the causative role played by psychological stress and vocal abuse among other factors and suggests speech therapy as being useful.

Therapy for ventricular phonation is similar to that for overcoming functional misphonia. The pitch must invariably be raised to an optimal or supraoptimal pitch level, and the tone focus must be changed from laryngopharyngeal resonance to nasopharyngeal resonance initially and then modified to naso-oropharyngeal resonance. Exercises to accomplish this have been described previously. The prognosis for ventricular phonation may vary from guarded to good, depending upon the individual patient, how long the problem has been in existence, how much need the patient has for this voice, and other related factors. A review of our cases experiencing ventricular phonation reveals the following information regarding the patients seen, the length of treatment and the results, as well as percentages of the information.

From Charts 5 and 6, the following conclusions may be drawn:

1. Of the 11 patients seen, 6 or 54.5 percent entered therapy.

2. Of the 6 patients entering therapy, 3 or 50 percent completed therapy.

3. Of the 3 patients completing therapy, 1 or 33.3 percent had long-term therapy and 2 or 66.7 percent had short-term therapy.

4. Of the 3 patients completing therapy, the results were excellent, 2 or 66.7 percent; good, 1 or 33.3 percent.

5. The comparison between males and females seen: males, 4 or 36.4 percent; females, 7 or 63.6 percent.

6. The inconclusive patients (3) for this dysphonia had all received long-term therapy, which is very unusual. Most inconclusives are short-term, usually less than six sessions or one month of therapy.

HYSTERICAL APHONIA, HYSTERICAL DYSPHONIA, AND FUNCTIONAL APHONIA

Three feasible categories have been observed in patients originally referred as hysterical aphonia. These categories are functional aphonia, hysterical aphonia, and hysterical dysphonia. Some authors use the terms functional aphonia and hysterical aphonia interchangeably; however, this author prefers to distinguish between the two. Functional aphonia refers to a voice loss without a psychological causation and usually with little or no psychological reaction to the loss of voice. Hysterical aphonia or dysphonia refers to a voice loss or an impaired voice with or without a psychological causation but with a marked psychological reaction to the loss of voice. For example, a cold which creates a loss of voice is not a psychological causation; however, the psychological reaction to the lack of voice can result in hysterical aphonia.

Hysterical aphonia and dysphonia are essentially psychological disorders or reactions. The term aphonia refers to the complete absence of voice; a whisper is used. Dysphonia is an impaired voice.

From clinical experience, in functional aphonia, the loss of voice may be due to vocal misuse or abuse, to an upper respiratory infection or cold, to laryngeal surgery, or injury to the laryngeal area. Functional aphonia occurs when a loss of voice exists in a larynx which has returned to a normal condition following laryngeal surgery or injury; if the larynx is impaired, the problem is not functional. In this grouping, the individual has little or no psychological reaction to the loss of voice. However, if the problem remains for more than a brief period of time, it may progress into hysterical aphonia or hysterical dysphonia as the individual begins to react or to react more severely to his lack of voice.

The initiating causes of hysterical aphonia and dysphonia are psychological trauma, physiological trauma, a cold or virus infection, or vocal misuse, the latter three being followed by a noticeable psychological reaction. Examples of psychological trauma are automobile accidents (without injury), divorce, separation, family conflicts, religious conflicts, personal problems involving the family, school, job, or friends, death of a relative or an important person to the individual, or any problem other than physical to which the individual reacts psychologically by a loss or an impairment of voice. Examples of physiological trauma which may be followed by a psychological reaction are (1) surgical procedures on the laryngeal area (including intubation) or accidents with injury to the laryngeal or pharyngeal area, such as whiplash in a car accident, a blow to the neck during swimming, surfing, ball games, or other activities, attempted strangulation and inhalation of smoke or chemical fumes; and (2) surgical procedures or accidents affecting other parts of the body.

In both hysterical aphonia and dysphonia, the physiological trauma, if affecting the laryngeal area in any degree, has had no permanent effect on this area; the larynx is essentially normal, but the marked psychological reaction from the physiological trauma creates the hysterical aphonia or dysphonia. The larynx is also essentially normal in functional aphonia; this category differs from hysterical aphonia following laryngeal surgery or injury, upper respiratory infection, or vocal misuse in that the patient has little or no psychological reaction to the laryngeal trauma. In other words, if the individual reacts severely to the loss or impairment of voice or if he deliberately cultivates the voice impairment after the larynx has returned to normal following laryngeal surgery or injury, infection, or vocal misuse, the diagnosis is hysterical aphonia or dysphonia. If the loss or impairment of voice is considered normal following laryngeal trauma and the individual shows little or no reaction, the problem is functional aphonia.

Regarding the incidence of functional aphonia, Brodnitz (1969, p. 1245) writes:

> Of 2,087 cases of all forms of voice disorders seen by the author, 1,677 or 80 percent belonged to the group of voice impairments that are not caused by a primary organic handicap. Of these cases, 74 or 4.4 percent were diagnosed as functional aphonia.

Lell (1941) reports that the most outstanding etiological factor of functional aphonia is an acute inflammatory process in or near the larynx. Aronson *et al.* (1964, p. 379) in studying 20 patients with the diagnoses of hysterical or conversion aphonia and dysphonia report:

> None of the patients had histories of emotional or physical trauma associated with the voice disorder. Patients from all four groups had

symptoms of cold or flu preceding onset of their voice disorder. . . .
Most of the patients in groups I, II, and III experienced fatigue or
exhaustion associated with the onset of their voice symptoms.

They also note that the onset of whispered speech was abrupt
in some, while in others the symptom of hoarseness was present
previously.

Hysterical aphonia and dysphonia afford sufficient secondary
gains that require understanding and appreciation. These conditions may be amply rewarding to the individual for him to initiate and/or maintain the voice disorder. The patient may be ac-
corded sympathy, allowed privileges, given attention, and removed from an unpleasant situation, such as a job or position
he dislikes. Thus, a seemingly negative condition becomes a
positive asset. Despite the negative vocal image presented by
the problems in communication, the motivating factors for the
onset and continuation are strong enough to perpetuate the
aphonia or dysphonia.

Aronson *et al.* (1966, p. 126-127), in studying 27 patients, ar-
rive at the following conclusions:

> 1. Acute and chronic situational conflicts were causally related to
> the voice disorders in the overwhelming majority of patients, regard-
> less of type of voice symptomatology.
> 2. The voice symptoms served the function of primary gain in
> that they resolved the situational conflict at least temporarily. Sec-
> ondary gain in the form of attention and sympathy from others was
> also noted in a large percentage of patients.
>
> . . . .
>
> 4. No serious psychopathology warranting immediate psychiatric
> help was found in any patient in this study.

Bangs and Freidinger (1949, 1950) outline therapy programs
for hysterical aphonia and hysterical dysphonia. Boone (1966)
describes two cases of functional aphonia which were treated
by symptomatic voice therapy and strong psychological support.
Wolski and Wiley (1965) recommend voice therapy plus psychiatric treatment for functional aphonia. Barton (1960) notes
the whispering syndrome of hysterical dysphonia and recommends treatment by psychoanalysis. Aronson (1969) has successfully removed symptoms by voice therapy in 39 of 40 patients

with psychogenic aphonia. He (p. 341) presents transcripts of three cases to show among other things, "the inseparability of voice therapy from the emotional responses of the patient and the necessity for the clinician to deal with them in the context of voice-symptom therapy." Brodnitz (1969), in discussing functional aphonia, cites vocal recovery for 51 out of 53 patients, with 44 patients recovering the voice during the first session; the other patients needed additional attempts. He (pp. 1251-1252) continues: "On the average, four to six sessions were required to stabilize the recovered voice at a normal level of loudness and resonance, to discuss the background of the disease and to decide on the need for psychotherapy."

Vocal rehabilitation for patients with functional aphonia is similar to that previously described for functional misphonia. Hysterical aphonia and dysphonia requires a therapist who is knowledgeable in psychotherapy as well as vocal rehabilitation. Hysterical aphonia and dysphonia may be temporary and transitory, disappearing without professional assistance. When these conditions are intermittent or chronic, therapy is appropriate.

To reestablish the voice in therapy, the following exercises are recommended. All of these therapy steps may be experienced in one session; however, not all steps are necessary for each patient.

The patient may be able to vocalize the "um-hum" because the lips are closed and because it is a mechanical sound and not threatening to the patient. The patient must be reassured that sound still exists. The patient is directed to vocalize "um-hum," "nim," or "me" from the lowest to the highest pitch levels and from the highest down to the lowest. Additional exercises, "me-me one" or "nim-nim one" or "um-hum one" (to ten), are used at approximately the optimal pitch level or where the voice is the fullest and easiest. Gentle effort and moderate volume is essential. Voice breaks often occur in these early stages of therapy; the patient is told this is to be expected.

Additional methods to initiate the voice may be based upon the cough, such as a gentle cough followed by verbalizing a number, "(cough), one," "(cough), two." Another method is having the patient assume another position, such as lying supine on a couch, and vocalizing a vowel /o/, /u/ or /i/ from the bottom to the top and back to the bottom of the pitch range.

After the patient has mastered the sound in mechanical exercises, the voice is transferred from the exercises to words, using either word lists or words the patient wishes to use. When the patient is able to carry over the sound from the mechanical exercises to the word, the words are spoken on different pitch levels so as to reestablish the patient's total pitch range. The words are followed by phrases and sentences, either reading these from a book or speaking spontaneously.

In the vast majority of patients, the patient is not told the condition is psychological; a more physiological approach is taken. The patient is told that he is having difficulty because the voice has not been used for a while or that it has been misused and abused. Some patients later require information regarding the psychological aspects of the problem. Vocal psychotherapy or psychotherapy is needed for these patients so that the problem will not recur.

The problem can be resolved within one or two therapy sessions, but it may require three to six months for a complete resolution. If the therapist feels that the patient is not responding to therapy and vocal psychotherapy after a reasonable period of time, the patient is referred for psychotherapy.

The causes of the dysphonias seen by this author are as follows:

Hysterical Aphonia		*Hysterical Dysphonia*		*Functional Aphonia*	
Death	2	Shock	1	Cold	4
Surgery	1	Holdup	1	Thyroiditis	1
Death wish	1	Emotional conflict	1		
Accident	1	Vocal misuse	6		
Homesickness	1				
Schizophrenia	1				
Vocal misuse	1				
Emotional conflict	1				

From Charts 7 and 8, the following conclusions may be drawn regarding hysterical aphonia:

1. Of the 9 patients seen, 5 or 55.6 percent entered therapy.

2. Of the 5 patients entering therapy, 4 or 80 percent completed therapy.

3. Of the 4 patients completing therapy, 4 or 100 percent had short-term therapy.

4. Of the 4 patients completing therapy, the results were excellent, 3 or 75 percent; good, 1 or 25 percent.

5. The comparison between males and females seen: males, 1 or 11.1 percent; females, 8 or 88.9 percent.

From Charts 9 and 10, the following conclusions may be drawn regarding hysterical dysphonia:

1. Of the 9 patients seen, 6 or 66.7 percent entered therapy.

2. Of the 6 patients entering therapy, 6 or 100 percent completed therapy.

3. Of the 6 patients completing therapy, 1 or 16.7 percent had long-term therapy and 5 or 83.3 percent had short-term therapy.

4. Of the 6 patients completing therapy, the results were excellent, 4 or 66.7 percent; good 2 or 33.3 percent.

5. The comparison between males and females seen: males, 2 or 22.2 percent; females, 7 or 77.8 percent.

From Charts 11 and 12, the following conclusions may be drawn regarding functional aphonia:

1. Of the 5 patients seen, 5 or 100 percent entered therapy.

2. Of the 5 patients entering therapy, 5 or 100 percent completed therapy.

3. Of the 5 patients completing therapy, 5 or 100 percent had short-term therapy.

4. Of the 5 patients completing therapy, the results were excellent, 5 or 100 percent.

5. The comparison between males and females seen: males, 1 or 20 percent; females, 4 or 80 percent.

SPASTIC DYSPHONIA AND INCIPIENT SPASTIC DYSPHONIA

Spastic dysphonia is a functional voice disorder in which the voice sounds "strangled." Incipient spastic dysphonia (Cooper, 1970b), a less severe form of spastic dysphonia, is often a forerunner of spastic dysphonia. Incipient spastic dysphonia had preceded spastic dysphonia in nearly all cases of spastic dysphonia seen. Both conditions should be treated by vocal rehabilitation and vocal psychotherapy, plus psychotherapy if necessary.

In spastic dysphonia and incipient spastic dysphonia, the pitch level is usually the basal or near basal pitch level for both males and females. The tone focus is often within the laryngopharynx. The volume is minimal during the episodes of vocal disability. In approximately 10 percent of the cases seen, the pitch level was too high.

Incipient spastic dysphonia and spastic dysphonia, like stuttering, are variable in their symptomatology. The negative vocal symptoms are voice skips, voice breaks, missed speech sounds, temporary loss of voice during conversation, inappropriate change in pitch, in quality, and/or in volume, neck muscle cording, tension or tightness in the throat, a choking sensation, effortful voice, reduced vocal range, and inability to talk voluntarily and at length in variable situations. The essential symptomatology as defined above recurs often for almost all patients. Some individuals report a clear voice upon arising in the morning while others deny this state. Many note the voice is clear at variable times with different people but with no consistent, definitive pattern prevailing.

Although these symptoms are similar in both conditions, the symptoms in incipient spastic dysphonia are much less severe, occur less frequently, and create much less emotional trauma. The extent of the spastic condition, its stage, and its severity may be indexed by the severity and frequency of the symptoms as well as the number of situations and people which produce the condition.

In spastic dysphonia, the episodes of spasticity are more protracted than they are in incipient spastic dysphonia, and the attempted control of spastic dysphonia by the individual becomes more demanding and more disabling. The spasticity of the vocal folds, which initially produces the condition, becomes more pervasive and more encompassing. Additional intrinsic laryngeal muscles, other than the vocal folds, and the extrinsic laryngeal and pharyngeal musculature become involved. Extreme tension of the chest and abdominal muscles is often common in well-established cases of spastic dysphonia.

The etiology of spastic dysphonia is currently in dispute, but the preponderance of the literature relative to this condition underscores psychological trauma as the basic cause. Bloch (1965), Heaver (1959, 1960), and Arnold (1959) are proponents of the psychological position for the etiological causation and recommend psychiatric treatment plus vocal rehabilitation. Robe, Brumlik, and Moore (1960) and Aronson *et al.* (1968a, 1968b) have indicated the neurological aspects of the disorder. Bicknell, Greenhouse, and Pesch (1968) favor a neurogenic or physiological disturbance as the origin and recommend investigation of conditioned reflex therapy.

This author posits the onset and development of incipient spastic dysphonia and spastic dysphonia are due to long-term vocal misuse with psychological or physical trauma often being the catalyst. The psychological factor may be an accident, a death, a divorce, loss of job or position, or any incident which emotionally affects the individual and which is reflected in his voice, creating a dysphonia. The psychological trauma need not be of an immediate nature. It may well be protracted internal or external emotional tensions, such as the inability to handle a job, feelings of inadequacy, and personality insecurity, among other factors. Individuals who have been diagnosed as having spastic dysphonia due to a specific accident or incident, such as a car mishap, have often been found to have had well defined incipient spastic dysphonia prior to any such incident. Physical trauma may involve a cold or upper respiratory problem, a long or severe illness, or surgery. These physical factors may influence the larynx directly, such as infecting the area, and create vocal misuse, or they may influence the vocal folds indirectly, such as creating physical fatigue or emotional depression, and may lead to vocal misuse through a lowered pitch of voice usually and laryngopharyngeal tone focus. As in ventricular phonation, the patient may prefer this altered voice and continue to use it.

Incipient spastic dysphonia may remain as such for a number of years. A situation(s) that is traumatic to the individual with this condition or continued vocal misuse may move the condition to the established and fully recognized state easily identified as spastic dysphonia. The incipient stage of spastic dysphonia often appears to be overlooked and misdiagnosed by physicians and speech therapists. Patients experiencing incipient spastic dysphonia and complaining of vocal disability and negative vocal symptoms may be afforded one or more of the palliative treatments. If a thorough medical examination requiring extensive testing is negative, the physician may advise a further checkup in a year or so if the patient still has the problem. Ferguson (1955, p. 331) observes:

> One needs a practiced ear to recognize the early stage of spastic dysphonia, before organic damage is evident and to sense the true cause of the strained, tired neck and chest muscles, or of the vague discomforts these patients relate to the throat and neck. Even in later stages when diffuse traumatic laryngitis is present, it is often difficult to separate or to distinguish cause from effect. Many such illnesses have been treated vigorously by antibiotic drugs and by voice rest, and most, if not all, have promptly recurred when the rest period ended. All cases of chronic or frequently recurring laryngitis should be suspected of vocal trauma.

A case in point is that of a young executive who experienced voice disability following a cold and was afforded numerous medical examinations and treatment and psychiatric assistance, all of which failed to halt the progressive vocal deterioration. The patient progressed from incipient spastic dysphonia to spastic dysphonia within five years. The frequency and duration of the dysphonia extended to almost all situations and circumstances, as contrasted to the incipient stage when the condition was contained to specific situations and circumstances. This case is not unique nor is it isolated. The therapy results for this individual are good.

Individuals react with different dysphonias to continued vocal misuse and physical or psychological trauma. Incipient spastic dysphonia and spastic dysphonia are only two dysphonic conditions. Others include hysterical aphonia, hysterical dysphonia, and ventricular phonation. An individual may progress through several of the dysphonic stages, such as incipient spastic dysphonia to spastic dysphonia, or from one condition to another, such as hysterical aphonia to spastic dysphonia. A young lady who was trapped in a fire developed hysterical aphonia which progressed to ventricular phonation and eventuated in incipient spastic dysphonia. The incipient spastic dysphonia was overcome within a year through vocal rehabilitation.

Many people commit vocal misuse without realizing it physically or mentally and yet never develop spastic dysphonia. The susceptibility of the individual to spastic dysphonia can be accounted for by the extent and frequency of vocal misuse, the extent and duration of psychological trauma, and physiological stability of the laryngeal mechanism to withstand vocal trauma, and the ability and willingness of the individual to confront psychological trauma by adjusting to the situation and not allowing such trauma to be reflected in the laryngeal mechanism and voice.

The factors responsible for some individuals being vulnerable to spastic dysphonia are also responsible for the extension and continuance of the spasticity. To undo a spastic voice of any degree requires willingness to face and deal with the vocal and psychological factors contributing to it. For some patients experiencing incipient spastic dysphonia or spastic dysphonia, these conditions are crutches which remove them from the responsibilities, problems, or anxieties which they must face. The case histories of patients with these conditions are replete with numerous statements of disability, disengagement, and disavowal of situations, circumstances, and people they must encounter, including their self-confrontation within these situations. Of all the voice disorders caused by vocal misuse and/or psychological or physical trauma, incipient spastic dysphonia and spastic dysphonia are the most severely involving and disabling. The patient with spastic dysphonia (less so with incipient spastic dysphonia) often refuses to accept the disorder as stemming from vocal disability and psychological trauma and fails to willingly confront himself in regard to the existence and continuance of the problem.

The treatment of incipient spastic dysphonia requires competent vocal therapy and vocal psychotherapy. Spastic dysphonia also requires vocal rehabilitation and vocal psychotherapy but often requires psychotherapy as well. Hypnosis was not of assistance to those patients who attempted this type of treatment. As previously mentioned, one case of spastic dysphonia was caused by self-hypnosis.

Vocal rehabilitation for incipient spastic dysphonia and spastic dysphonia is the same. As in all voice problems, the need to locate and establish the optimal pitch is vital. It has been found that some patients respond well to the supraoptimal pitch level and then are able to redefine the pitch level to the optimal pitch level. Most spastic dysphonia patients seen need to have the pitch raised and the tone focus changed from the laryngopharynx to a balanced oronasolaryngopharyngeal resonance. Most patients whose pitch is too high are brought down in pitch to the optimal pitch level. A few may need the basal or near basal range, as discussed in falsetto voice, before finding optimal range.

The same exercises that are utilized for developing optimal pitch level and range for functional misphonia is applicable for this condition. Midsection breath support is vital for these patients as they are frequently tensing and constricting upper chest and midsection musculature as well as pharyngeal and laryngeal musculature. The volume should be minimized not only during therapy but also following the completion of therapy. The spasticity of the vocal folds is activated by habituated immoderate or habituated excessive volume. Some patients respond to the use of a breathy voice quality which eliminates the choking or forcing. Fox (1969) cites the use of a breathy voice in the one case reported.

Many similarities exist between spastic dysphonia and stuttering. The spastic dysphonic has a vocal image which is a counterpart to that of the speech image of the secondary stutterer. The belief and feeling that vocalization is ever uncertain adds to the trauma of the vocal disorder itself. Spastic dysphonia is similar to stuttering in that there is an approach-avoidance process (Sheehan, 1970) also in spastic dysphonia which has been fashioned and solidified through the experiences of vocal disability. Role is an important factor in the ability or disability to speak, but it is a highly variable role process. Spastic dysphonics are variable in their ability to speak when alone and isolated. Some can sing clearly and easily; others cannot.

Once the condition of incipient spastic dysphonia is noticed, it must be identified and treated in the early stages. Incipient spastic dysphonia that has existed for a period of years has within its context and essence created extensive emotional concern and trauma. Despite these years of vocal trauma and emotional reaction to vocal trauma, the prognosis for incipient spastic dysphonia remains good to excellent. Like stuttering, this condition is more amenable to resolution in the incipient stage. Once the stage of spastic dysphonia is reached, the problem becomes one of first modifying and reducing the symptoms and then eliminating the problem entirely.

Spastic dysphonia has one of the worse prognoses of all voice disorders. It presents the greatest extent of vocal disability due to the uncertainty of pitch, volume, quality, and tone focus. It also holds the least chance for elimination due to the circular effect (spastic speech to emotional reaction to continued spasticity, and so on), and due to a number of complex contributory factors (vocal misuse, vocal image). Both the circular effect and the contributory factors become more severe with the continuance of the condition. Spastic dysphonia requires the greatest amount of vocal retraining and vocal psychotherapy to change the vocal image of all vocal disabilities. The prognosis for spastic dysphonia is guarded to fair in most patients. In patients who are fully cooperative and are willing to undergo therapy for two to three years, the prognosis is good and, in a few cases, excellent.

Spastic dysphonia has been described in the literature as rare or infrequent in incidence. Of 1406 cases seen involving voice disorders over the past ten years, approximately 4.5 percent would be classified as incipient spastic dysphonia and spastic dysphonia. This percentage should not be considered rare or infrequent. The lack of identification of this disorder may well contribute to this erroneous designation.

Of the 42 spastic dysphonia and the 21 incipient spastic dysphonic patients seen, the causes of the dysphonias are as follows:

Spastic Dysphonia

Death (husband)	5	Incest	1
Cold	4	Accident	1
Surgery	3	Alcoholism	1
Divorce	2	Business failure	1
Son in Vietnam	2	Emotional conflict	10
Flood	1	Vocal misuse	10
Self hypnosis	1		

Incipient Spastic Dysphonia

Holdup 2	Plane crash 1
Surgery 1	Inefficient vocal therapy
Accident 1	(incorrect pitch level) 1
Fire 1	Emotional conflict 7
Interracial marriage 1	Vocal misuse 5
Death (wife) 1	

Charts 13-16 indicate the age of the patients, the length of time in therapy, the results, and the percentages of each.

From Charts 13 and 14, the following conclusions may be drawn regarding spastic dysphonia:

1. Of the 42 patients seen, 22 or 52.4 percent entered therapy.

2. Of the 22 patients entering therapy, 6 or 27.3 percent completed therapy.

3. Of the 6 patients completing therapy, 6 or 100 percent had long-term therapy.

4. Of the 6 patients completing therapy, the results were excellent, 1 or 16.7 percent; good, 3 or 50 percent; fair, 2 or 33.3 percent.

5. The comparison between males and females seen: males, 18 or 42.9 percent; females, 24 or 57.1 percent.

6. Of the 16 inconclusive patients, 4 were long-term inconclusive.

From Charts 15 and 16, the following conclusions may be drawn regarding incipient spastic dysphonia:

1. Of the 21 patients seen, 13 or 61.9 percent entered therapy.

2. Of the 13 patients entering therapy, 9 or 69.2 percent completed therapy.

3. Of the 9 patients completing therapy, 3 or 33.3 percent had long-term therapy and 6 or 66.7 percent had short-term therapy.

4. Of the 9 patients completing therapy, the results were excellent, 6 or 66.7 percent; good, 2 or 22.2 percent; fair, 1 or 11.1 percent.

5. The comparison between males and females seen: males, 7 or 33.3 percent; females, 14 or 66.7 percent.

NASALITY

Nasality is created by too much nasal resonance. Moser, Dreher, and Alder (1955) note that hypernasality is detrimental to intelligibility. Diehl and McDonald (1956, p. 237) find: "Only simulated breathy and nasal qualities appear to interfere with communication."

Vocal rehabilitation is recommended for nasality in most cases. Brodnitz (1963, p. 155) writes: "All patients with permanent *hypernasality* profited greatly from voice therapy." Adler (1960), in treating hypernasality, uses kinesthetic and visual awareness of tongue, vocal phonics, louder voice, and breath control, among other techniques. Sherman and Goodwin (1954) are opposed to lowering the pitch level as a routine technique for treating hypernasality. From this author's clinical experience lowering the pitch was necessary in nearly all cases.

Nasality may be functional, organic (structural), or neurological in etiology. The majority of patients seen with nasality were functional in nature. Functional nasality may be caused by imitation of a poor vocal model, lack of vocal training, or a vocal image. Functional nasality is often amenable to vocal rehabilitation; organic nasality may be amenable; neurological nasality, such as that created by myasthenia gravis, may not be. (Hypernasality may be a symptom of myasthenia gravis, according to Wolski [1967].)

Clinical experience with neurologically created nasality, such as that following a surgical procedure relating to brain function or to a stroke, discloses unpredictable results. Some cases improve spontaneously. One female patient was hospitalized with the diagnosis of neurological impairment and extremely hypernasal speech. The voice spontaneously recovered within a period of a few months.

Organic nasality, such as that created by cleft palate, is responsive to vocal rehabilitation, if the program of therapy begins early enough under competent direction and there is carry-over in the home. It is also important to have vocal therapy early in order to habituate the child to a new vocal image and a new vocal identity as well as to a new vocal pattern. The child with a cleft palate can benefit by utilizing the basic principles of the exercises described in this section, if they are modified and combined with play therapy; however, the child must have additional articulation and language therapy which is not covered in this book.

Tonsillectomies and adenoidectomies may contribute to the onset and development of hypernasality in some patients. In a few cases, an insufficient amount of pharyngeal tissue may remain following an adenoidectomy and/or a short palate may exist so that the individual is unable to achieve closure; the prognosis in these few cases is guarded. In others, the pharyngeal area may be sensitized by the surgical procedure so that the individual does not compensate for the removal of tissue. The hypernasality created in these cases is more amenable to therapy if treated shortly after the surgery. However, clinical experience indicates that parents are often assured that the child will outgrow the problem. The longer the problem remains, the more trying and difficult is the resolution. Nonetheless, the prognosis remains good to excellent for these cases whether the hypernasality is of long or of short duration.

Since nasality is created by excessive nasal resonance, it is desirous to alter the balance of tone focus from the nasopharynx to the oropharynx. The danger inherent in such an approach is that the patient may develop too much laryngopharyngeal resonance in the process of changing the nasal resonance. When the tone focus is changed from nasal resonance to a more dominant oral resonance so that the oral and nasal resonance is balanced, the pitch of voice is often concomitantly lowered. It is essential to locate the optimal pitch level for the individual experiencing nasality. In some cases, it may be more appropriate to seek the lowest pitch within the optimal pitch range so as to stress more oral resonance while avoiding the nasal resonance. Some individuals cannot establish or maintain the fine balance of oral and nasal resonance that defines a so-called normal voice. These individuals are afforded more oral resonance so that they can more easily determine the difference between oral and nasal resonance. Other individuals experiencing nasality may benefit from a more breathy tonal quality with concomitantly less carrying power to the voice. The breathy tone is more acceptable to our society than is the nasality. A young lady of fourteen years of age was quite agreeable to a breathy voice because it was an acceptable tone and voice to her sisters and to her classmates.

Exercises to Eliminate Nasality

Relevant exercises specific to removing nasality begin with vowels which stress oral resonance, such as /o/ and /u/.

1. The /o/ is produced repeatedly by the patient, using the lowest level of the optimal pitch range, until the sound is acceptable to the therapist as oral in resonance. The exercise is recorded on Language Master cards, is played back after each attempt, and is evaluated by the therapist. For instance, the patient repeats /o/ for the length of the recording of the Language Master card, a matter of six seconds. Then the card is played back with the therapist counseling or advising the patient regarding the acceptability of the sound. Modification of the sound is made over a period of therapy sessions until the pitch and tone focus on the vowel /o/ is acceptable to the therapist. Key cards are then made of this sound or tone and kept to be used during the following session. These cards may be given to the patient if he has a Language Master at home to use for reference during practice between therapy sessions. The first vowel is the most difficult to master, since the patient has no criteria except that which the therapist tells him. From the mastery of the first vowel, the patient begins to get auditory and kinesthetic feedback and is able to practice the vowel sound outside of therapy; the vowel /o/ is not necessarily the first vowel to begin with, as some patients find the /u/ more amenable to control.

2. When the patient is able to master one vowel, he is afforded a second vowel, such as /u/. The above process is repeated. During the mastery of the second vowel, the patient uses the first vowel and the reference or key card as a guide for the mastery of the second vowel. The mastery of the sounds is not smooth nor consistent. Therapy consists of progress, plateau, and regression.

After a number of sessions, a vowel may be controlled most of the time with the percentage of improvement occurring more rapidly as the sessions progress. With both the first and second vowels, regression of the control of the correct vowel resonance occurs from session to session as well as within each session.

3. Numbers, such as "/o/-one, /o/-two," are added to the vowel when mastery of the vowel alone occurs. It is vital that the patient master one vowel at a time so that he can produce the "/o/-one, /o/-two" (to ten) correctly before moving to the second vowel. He then moves to "/u/-one, /u/-two" (to ten).

4. The next step involves combinations of vowels, such as "/o/-/u/-one, /o/-/u/-two" (to ten). This combination of vowels is more involved and more demanding of the patient's ability to monitor and produce the correct sound.

5. When mastery of the vowel combinations and numbers occur, this is followed by single words, such as "/o/-/u/-one, hello," "/o/-/u/-one, house." These words are taken from word lists, so that the patient is able to concentrate on the sound and need not concern himself with selecting a spontaneous sound. The single word practice is followed by phrase practice, such as "/o/-/u/-one, hello there," "/o/-/u/-two, only tomorrow."

6. Sentences are finally used, such as "/o/-/u/-one, the sun is setting tomorrow." Again, as with single words, the phrases and sentences are usually taken from a book.

7. Spontaneous speech with an oral resonance is now the goal. The patient speaks spontaneously using one track of the Language Master card and compares this to the correctly produced vowel, number, and sentence combination on the other track of the card. The patient becomes his own therapist as he monitors the correct sound and tries to achieve it in spontaneous speech. The therapist continues to advise the patient when the sound is correctly or incorrectly produced.

The sequence of steps presented is not necessarily the approach with each patient. The therapist must determine for the patient the order and sequence of steps he must undergo. Patients vary in their ability to master a given vowel. With some patients it is necessary to establish oral resonance for all vowels before adding numbers to any vowel. The therapist must be the one to judge what vowel sequences are best for each patient and how much mastery of oral resonance via the vowels is necessary before proceeding to the next step. Some patients undergo abbreviated sequences of the previously mentioned exercises or skip entire segments of the programmed therapy regimen. Other patients quickly hear and establish the correct oral resonance; the therapist must move as rapidly as the patient is able to progress.

The problem of vocal identity and the vocal image is part of a total therapeutic approach. Since altering the voice may also change the personality, emotional and psychological considerations must be taken into account by vocal psychotherapy, or if necessary, psychotherapy as well.

With nasality it has been found relevant and instructive to afford associate therapy. For the adult, if married, the spouse is brought in. If the patient is unmarried, a close friend, a member of the family, or a secretary is appropriate to assist the patient outside of therapy. With children, usually the mother will suffice in carry-over from therapy session to the home or outside situation.

Patients who have nasality as a result of neurological etiology are included under Neurological Disorders. A review of cases of functional and organic nasality is found in Charts 17 through 20.

From Charts 17 and 18, the following conclusions may be drawn regarding functional nasality:

1. Of the 44 patients seen, 21 or 47.7 percent entered therapy.

2. Of the 21 patients entering therapy, 18 or 85.7 percent completed therapy.

3. Of the 18 patients completing therapy, 10 or 55.6 percent had long-term therapy and 8 or 44.4 percent had short-term therapy.

4. Of the 18 patients completing therapy, the results were excellent, 10 or 55.6 percent; good, 7 or 38.9 percent; fair, 1 or 5.6 percent.

5. The comparison between males and females seen: males, 23 or 52.3 percent; females, 21 or 47.7 percent.

6. The relatively high percentage of patients who were seen for evaluation only occurred because these patients were seen at a medical center and referred to speech therapists in their area for therapy.

From Charts 19 and 20, the following conclusions may be drawn regarding organic nasality:

1. Of the 11 patients seen, 7 or 63.6 percent entered therapy.

2. Of the 7 patients entering therapy, 7 or 100 percent completed therapy.

3. Of the 7 patients completing therapy, 5 or 71.4 percent had long-term therapy and 2 or 28.6 percent had short-term therapy.

4. Of the 7 patients completing therapy, the results were excellent, 3 or 42.8 percent; good, 3 or 42.8 percent; fair, 1 or 14.3 percent.

5. The comparison between males and females seen: males, 5 or 45.5 percent; females, 6 or 54.5 percent.

BOWED VOCAL FOLDS

The condition of bowed vocal folds as referred to in this book may be functional or organic in etiology. Bowed vocal folds that are functional in nature are created by vocal misuse and abuse and may be alleviated by vocal rehabilitation. Organic bowed vocal folds have an organic condition of nodules, polyps, or polypoid degeneration in addition to the bowing. Although surgery may be necessary prior to vocal rehabilitation to remove the organic lesions, especially polypoid degeneration, in some patients, the bowing and the growths (in other patients) are often amenable to vocal therapy.

Bowed vocal folds may be confused with two other dysphonic conditions which produce a noticeably breathy voice: paralytic dysphonia and myasthenia laryngis. In some cases of unilateral paralytic dysphonia, the paralyzed cord is bowed in the midline position or in the paramedian position. If the paralyzed fold is in the midline position, vocal rehabilitation alone is often successful. If the cord is in the paramedian position, a Teflon injection followed by vocal rehabilitation may be necessary, if vocal rehabilitation alone is unsuccessful (see Paralytic Dysphonia).

Myasthenia laryngis is a term used by Jackson (1940, p. 434) to describe "a morbid entity characterized by asthenia of the phonatory musculature of the larynx, especially the powerful overworked thyroarytenoideus muscles." Jackson considers myasthenia laryngis as a muscular disability. He posits a continuum of this condition, with the possibility of controlling the early stages through extended vocal rest and proper vocal training. He (p. 461) adds: "that cure is obtainable only in the earlier stages of the disease." According to Jackson, myasthenia laryngis is created by too high a pitch in singing and in speaking; vocal abuse is the chief etiological factor.

Differential diagnosis between myasthenia laryngis and unilateral paralytic dysphonia in the intermediate (cadaveric) position cannot be made auditorily by the voice therapist. A similar auditory presentation, leakage of air and effortful voice, is afforded to the voice therapist by these two conditions. Unilateral paralytic dysphonia with the cord in the paramedian position may also resemble myasthenia laryngis auditorily, but an effortful volume at the optimal pitch level may reveal a natural voice. Myasthenia laryngis in the final stage does not present a discernible optimal pitch nor a clear tone. The voice quality is noticeably breathy.

When the vocal fold is paralyzed in the midline position or if the patient is in the first stage of myasthenia laryngis, the patient's production of the optimal pitch level as directed by the voice therapist may immediately result in a clear and normal voice. A program of vocal rehabilitation must be undertaken to maintain the optimal pitch.

The voice therapist may be able to determine if the patient has temporarily bowed vocal folds (functional or organic) or myasthenia laryngis in the final stage. If the patient is able to laugh at his optimal pitch level with a clear tone that is not breathy, the patient has bowed vocal folds. If the sound continues to be breathy when the patient is using the optimal pitch level, then myasthenia laryngis may be present.

In this final stage of myasthenia laryngis, the vocal folds may be bowed, but they respond minimally to maximal vocal rehabilitation. The condition of bowed vocal folds (functional or organic) may be considered to be on a continuum leading to myasthenia laryngis (first stage and second stage) if vocal misuse is persistent.

Wilson (1966, p. 79) recommends lowering the habitual pitch for bowed cords: "In addition, it is often necessary to eliminate vocal abuse such as loud talking and yelling, to establish correct pitch usage often by lowering the habitual level, and to improve the clarity of the voice." Clinical experience with 42 patients with bowed vocal folds is entirely contrary to this point of view; almost all of these patients had been using too low a pitch level. Raising the pitch of voice for these patients as well as increasing the oronasal resonance eliminated the bowing and created an efficient voice.

Vocal therapy for bowed vocal folds is similar to that used for paralytic dysphonia in which the paralyzed cord is in the median position; the therapy is described under Paralytic Dysphonia. (See Charts 21 through 24 for functional and organic bowed vocal folds.)

From Charts 21 and 22, the following conclusions may be drawn regarding bowed vocal folds—functional:

1. Of the 32 patients seen, 26 or 81.25 percent entered therapy.

2. Of the 26 patients entering therapy, 24 or 92.3 percent completed therapy.

3. Of the 24 patients completing therapy, 7 or 29.2 percent had long-term therapy and 17 or 70.8 percent had short-term therapy.

4. Of the 24 patients completing therapy, the results were excellent, 20 or 83.3 percent; good, 2 or 8.3 percent; fair, 2 or 8.3 percent.

5. The comparison between males and females seen: males, 20 or 62.5 percent; females, 12 or 37.5 percent.

From Charts 23 and 24, the following conclusions may be drawn regarding bowed vocal folds—organic:

1. Of the 10 patients seen, 10 or 100 percent entered therapy.

2. Of the 10 patients entering therapy, 7 or 70 percent completed therapy.

3. Of the 7 patients completing therapy, 3 or 42.9 percent had long-term therapy and 4 or 57.1 percent had short-term therapy.

4. Of the 7 patients completing therapy, the results were excellent, 5 or 71.4 percent; good, 2 or 28.6 percent.

5. The comparison between males and females seen: males, 3 or 30 percent; females, 7 or 70 percent.

6. Of the 10 patients seen, in addition to the bowing, 7 had nodules (5 no surgery; 2 postoperative), 1 had a polyp (1 postoperative), and 2 had polypoid degeneration (1 no surgery; 1 postoperative).

NODULES, POLYPS, AND POLYPOID DEGENERATION

Nodules and polyps, which are benign vocal fold growths may be unilateral or bilateral. Usually they are located on the anterior third of the vocal folds. Nodules are generally sessile; polyps are either sessile or pedunculated. The terms node and nodule are often used interchangeably. Polypoid degeneration is a series of, or extension of, polyps which may be located on a portion of the vocal fold or on the entire vocal fold, either unilaterally or bilaterally. Although laryngeal pain is usually associated with contact ulcer, patients with nodules and with polypoid degeneration have also complained of pain in this area.

The effect of vocal misuse and abuse on the causation of vocal fold nodules, polyps, and polypoid degeneration has been previously discussed. The total treatment program, including the appropriateness of a surgical procedure, has also been included. Some postsurgical patients who have undergone unilateral or bilateral stripping of the vocal folds for polypoid degeneration experience marked difficulty in securing or regaining a normal voice. A study by this author (1972), in comparing patients with nodules, polyps, and contact ulcers, found that the mean fundamental frequencies of postoperative groups (growth removed by surgery) were lower than the mean fundamental frequencies of no surgery groups (growth present; no surgery) both in males and in females prior to vocal rehabilitation.

Vocal therapy for these lesions is similar to the procedure previously outlined. Only one point needs further discussion because of the controversy which exists regarding the change of pitch in cases of vocal fold nodules. Some authors, such as Wilson (1966) and Van Riper and Irwin (1958), have recommended lowering the pitch usually. A review of this author's patients who had nodules as well as those patients having polyps and polypoid degeneration reveals that these patients had a long history of utilizing the basal or near basal pitch of voice. The pitch nearly always needed to be raised. In agreement are Fisher and Logemann (1970, p. 277) who report: "Our clinical experience has led to concurrence with Luchsinger and Arnold's observation of an unnaturally low speaking pitch in many nodule patients." They (p. 278) have also found: "Further, the case histories of many such patients suggested that use of an unnaturally low speaking pitch was a habit before the dysphonia began and might be credited, at least in part, with contributing to the development of the lesion." The vast majority of patients seen with nodules by this author were using the basal or near basal pitch of voice.

Nodules have been the most frequently seen organic condition. Luchsinger and Arnold (1965, p. 179) have also found: "The vocal nodule is the commonest chronic, though benign, laryngeal lesion removed surgically for diagnosis and therapy." The breakdown of the patients seen with nodules, polyps, and polypoid degeneration is shown on Charts 25 through 30.

From Charts 25 and 26, the following conclusions may be drawn regarding nodules:

1. Of the 254 patients seen, 190 or 74.8 percent entered therapy.

2. Of the 190 patients entering therapy, 178 or 93.7 percent completed therapy.

3. Of the 178 patients completing therapy, 48 or 27 percent had long-term therapy and 130 or 73 percent had short-term therapy.

4. Of the 178 patients completing therapy, the results were excellent, 125 or 70.2 percent; good, 29 or 16.3 percent; fair, 24 or 13.5 percent.

5. The comparison between males and females seen: males, 107 or 42.1 percent; females, 147 or 57.9 percent.

From Charts 27 and 28, the following conclusions may be drawn regarding polyps:

1. Of the 68 patients seen, 51 or 75 percent entered therapy.

2. Of the 51 patients entering therapy, 46 or 90.2 percent completed therapy.

3. Of the 46 patients completing therapy, 9 or 19.6 percent had long-term therapy and 37 or 80.4 percent had short-term therapy.

4. Of the 46 patients completing therapy, the results were excellent, 27 or 58.7 percent; good, 9 or 19.6 percent; fair, 10 or 21.7 percent.

5. The comparison between males and females seen: males, 25 or 36.8 percent; females, 43 or 63.2 percent.

From Charts 29 and 30, the following conclusions may be drawn regarding polypoid degeneration:

1. Of the 63 patients seen, 40 or 63.5 percent entered therapy.

2. Of the 40 patients entering therapy, 35 or 87.5 percent completed therapy.

3. Of the 35 patients completing therapy, 8 or 22.9 percent had long-term therapy and 27 or 77.1 percent had short-term therapy.

4. Of the 35 patients completing therapy, the results were excellent, 23 or 65.7 percent; good, 8 or 22.9 percent; fair, 4 or 11.4 percent.

5. The comparison between males and females seen: males, 12 or 19 percent; females, 51 or 81 percent.

CONTACT ULCERS

Jackson defined the condition of contact ulcer in 1928; however, Virchow referred to a condition similar to contact ulcer as "pachydermis laryngis" in 1858. Contact ulcer is a lesion which occurs on one or both of the medial surfaces of the arytenoid cartilages. In incipient contact ulcer, edema, inflammation, and/ or redness is present. As the contact ulcer develops, the interarytenoid area consists of "an area of exposed necrotic cartilage surrounded by a rim of raised granulation tissue" as described by Cooper and Nahum (1967, p. 41).

According to these authors (1967, p. 42), contact ulcer develops in three stages, the first stage being incipient contact ulcer:

The first stage is manifested by fatigue and hoarseness which occur at the end of the day or after periods of vocal stress. The amount of trauma required to produce the symptoms gradually decreases. Vocal rest, usually at night or on weekends or vacations, results in recovery and loss of the symptoms, but they recur more frequently as time goes on. Examination discloses minimal edema and redness of the interarytenoid area and is seen only when the patient has recently abused his voice. With rest the appearance returns to normal.

In the second stage there is continual hoarseness, fatigue, and occasional pain on speaking or swallowing, and rest affords only temporary relief. Examination shows severe inflammation with early loss

of the mucoperichondrium covering of the opposing arytenoid surfaces.

In the third stage there is severe constant hoarseness, fatigue, pain
on swallowing or talking, and little relief with the mere rest. Examination shows a denudation of the opposing cartilaginous surfaces
and a surrounding rim of granulation tissue.*

Since contact ulcer of the larynx is due mainly to vocal misuse and abuse, a major approach to the treatment is vocal rehabilitation. This disorder was initially treated by vocal rehabilitation by Peacher (1947c). Some authors have maintained that
emotional tension is the central cause of the contact ulcer.
Arnold (1966, p. 80) postulates: "Contact ulcer is a psychosomatic disease resulting from emotional tension." Peacher
(1961), in a follow-up of 70 cases, notes that superficial psychotherapy was adequate for most patients; only a small number
required psychotherapy. A review of this author's patients con-
firms Peacher's findings regarding psychotherapy. However, vocal psychotherapy was vital for all contact ulcer patients seen.

Jackson and Jackson (1935a) find that nearly all contact ulcer patients dated the onset of their laryngeal symptoms from
a cold or influenza. Holinger and Johnston (1960) also note that
26 patients out of 92 attributed the onset of the symptoms to
an acute upper respiratory condition.

Jackson and Jackson (1935a) warn that the condition is usually overlooked. Cooper and Nahum (1967) recommend that the
physician watch for the patient who is in the incipient or first
stage of contact ulcer. They (p. 42) continue:

Patients in the early stages are the easiest to treat and good results can be obtained relatively early, which prevents the long-term
problems associated with advanced cases.

Three different pathological conditions of contact ulcer have
been encountered. The first type is incipient contact ulcer,
which is treated by vocal rehabilitation alone. The second type
is the benign contact ulcer granuloma and/or fossa which is the
type that prevails most frequently. The granuloma may be treated by surgery prior to vocal rehabilitation; the fossa is usually
treated by vocal rehabilitation alone. The third type is the

---

* *Archives of Otolaryngology*, 85:42, 1967. Copyright 1967, American Medical
Association.

contact ulcer granuloma which has undergone malignant degeneration. This type is diagnosed by biopsy and treated by surgery and/or radiation followed possibly by vocal rehabilitation.

The treatment of contact ulcer by vocal rehabilitation affords excellent results. The usual duration of therapy falls within six to twelve months for a resolution of the lesion. A shorter period of time may eliminate the problem in some cases.

The contact ulcer patient is almost invariably at the basal or near basal pitch of voice. The tone focus is usually in the laryngopharynx. Poor vocal hygiene often accompanies the vocal misuse, adding to or initiating the condition itself. Therapy for this condition is the same as has been described.

Charts 31 and 32 describe the contact ulcer patients seen.

From Charts 31 and 32, the following conclusions may be drawn:

1. Of the 85 patients seen, 61 or 71.8 percent entered therapy.

2. Of the 61 patients entering therapy, 56 or 91.8 percent completed therapy.

3. Of the 56 patients completing therapy, 25 or 44.6 percent had long-term therapy and 31 or 55.4 percent had short-term therapy.

4. Of the 56 patients completing therapy, the results were excellent , 49 or 87.5 percent; good, 5 or 8.9 percent; fair, 2 or 3.6 percent.

5. The comparison between males and females seen: males, 66 or 77.6 percent; females, 19 or 22.4 percent.

PAPILLOMATOSIS

The etiology of papillomatosis remains obscure. Three major theories which attempt to explain the etiology of papillomatosis of the vocal folds are virus infection, hormonal imbalance, and trauma or vocal abuse and irritation.

Ullmann (1923) reports papilloma of the larynx was caused by a filterable virus. However, Ferguson and Scott (1944, p. 478) write: "Ullmann's series was small and poorly controlled, and his work has not been confirmed." Holinger, Schild, and Maurizi (1968, p. 1468) report:

> The results of many investigations point to viruses as the causal factor of papilloma. The evidence was thoroughly reviewed, but it

has not been possible to duplicate work previously reported on the presence of a species-specific virus capable of producing growth of tissue cultures with regrowth after blind serial tissue culture passes.

Regarding the influence of the endocrine system, Rubin (1954) and Baker (1965) note that papillomata in children may stop growing and may even disappear at puberty. Other authors, including Majoros, Parkhill, and Devine (1964) and Dekelboum (1965) do not find evidence to support this hormonal theory.

The theory of vocal misuse and abuse is discussed by Webb (1956, p. 877):

> Probably the earliest theory of etiology which still has its adherents is that expressed by Bosworth in 1892, and by Browne even earlier. They believed that papilloma of the larynx is the result of chronic irritation. Browne traced more than half of a series of 26 cases to overuse of the voice. More convincingly, in a series of 300 cases Fauvel found the greatest incidence among those whose work required special or excessive use of the voice, such as ministers.

Other authors who view chronic irritation or trauma as a possible etiological factor are Jackson (1960) and Dekelboum (1965) (adult papilloma). Vocal abuse, such as shouting and competing with noise, is evident in the case histories of many patients seen by this author.

The most common symptom of papillomata of the vocal folds is hoarseness. The lesion is generally located on the vocal fold, according to Shanks (1958, p. 219) "usually at or near the anterior third or at the anterior commissure." Ferguson and Scott (1944, p. 478) report: "The vocal cords are the most frequent sites, but the tumors may occur anywhere in the larynx." They continue: "In children, the lesions are usually multiple, as opposed to the more frequently single adult form."

Controversy exists as to the histopathological difference between childhood papillomata and adult papillomata. Although Bjork and Weber (1956) report a difference between laryngeal papillomata in the adult and in the child, Holinger, Schild, and Maurizi (1968), West, Boggs, and Holinger (1957), and Huizinga (1957) found no difference between the two types.

Types of treatment for laryngeal papillomata as listed by Holinger, Schild, and Maurizi (1968, pp. 1469-1472) are

1. Medical—topical and internal medications.

2. Immunological—vaccines.

3. Surgical procedures—forceps removal, tracheostomy, and thyrotomy.

4. Physical—thermal cautery, diathermy, radiation, cyro-surgery, and ultrasound.

These methods of treatment have had varying success; however, follow-up reports have not substantiated the early favorable results of these treatments. At the present, surgery, estradiol, vaccines, and ultrasound are the most frequently used treatments.

Szpunar (1967), in treating 107 patients with juvenile laryngeal papillomatosis, has had very good results in utilizing endoscopic removal and intralaryngeal injection of estradiol. Holinger, Schild, and Maurizi (1968) used an inactivated autogenous vaccine in 51 patients. Improvement was noted in 55 percent (28 patients); no change was observed in 25 percent (13 patients); 6 percent (3 patients) deteriorated; and adequate information was unavailable in 14 percent (7 patients). Ultrasound is discussed by Holinger, Schild, and Maurizi (1968, p. 1472):

> Undoubtedly the most significant new modality has been the use of ultrasound for the treatment of laryngeal papilloma.
>
> . . . .
>
> As with x-radiation, a final evaluation may not be possible for another 20 years. The effect of the ultrasound on nerve tissues and on the growth factors of the larynx is not known, and these important considerations cannot be ignored.

Radiation treatment for juvenile laryngeal papillomata has been found to be detrimental by Rabbett (1965) and Maier (1968).

Regarding the various types of treatment for laryngeal papillomatosis, Rosenbaum, Alavi, and Bryant (1968, p. 654) report:

> Some patients have undergone more than 100 procedures for removal of laryngeal papillomas. Many types of therapy, including steroids, sex hormones, Aureomycin, irradiation, and autogenous vaccines, have been employed. The long list of therapeutic agents indicates a lack of consistent results from any.

Despite the many medical approaches to the treatment of laryngeal papillomatosis, the dictum of Holinger, Schild, and Maurizi

(1968, p. 1462) remains: "Papilloma of the larynx continues to be an enigma."

Since vocal fold irritation is one of the three major theories for the etiology of papillomatosis of the vocal folds, it is surprising that vocal rehabilitation has not been a major means of treatment. Vocal rehabilitation for papillomatosis of the vocal folds has been attempted by Brodnitz (1963) and Cooper (1964, 1971a). Brodnitz found such therapy "helpful." A study begun in 1964 and completed in 1965 by Cooper (1971a) found that four of eight patients experiencing biopsied vocal fold papillomatosis revealed a reduction or a partial elimination of the condition following three months of vocal rehabilitation. Figure 1 indicates the extent of the condition prior to and following vocal rehabilitation.

A thorough discussion of these eight patients and comprehensive studies of the intensity, airflow rate, frequency, and quality, as well as an extended review of the literature can be found in Cooper (1964). The vocal therapy for papillomatosis is the same as therapy for other organic growths. A discussion of therapy is also included in Cooper (1971a). One point regarding pitch needs to be emphasized. The habitual pitch level may be too high in some patients, although it is generally too low in most patients. A vocal image usually exists in patients with papillomatosis.

Vocal rehabilitation is not always considered applicable nor relevant by physicians for the containment, reduction, and/or elimination of this condition. Therefore, few patients are available for study and review. A number of patients with papillomatosis made good to excellent progress in vocal rehabilitation in that there was a slight to extensive degree of reduction in the size and/or number of papillomata; however, by using the general criteria established for determining the therapy results (Part V), it was necessary to evaluate most patients as fair in that a portion of the growth remained. If the patients had remained in therapy for a longer period of time and had cooperated more fully in the program, it is believed that the final evaluation would have been good to excellent. Vocal rehabilitation should be an integral part of the treatment for vocal fold papillomatosis.

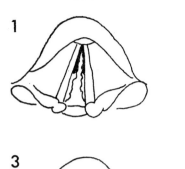
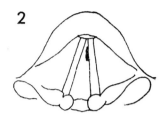
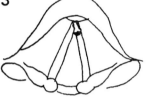
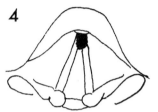
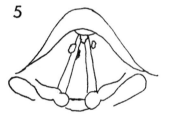
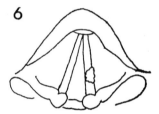
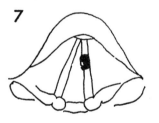
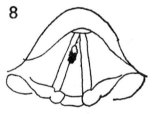

Figure 1. Papillomatosis before and after vocal rehabilitation. Before: outline of papillomata; after: black area. 1. Reduction, Female, age 10. Before: diffuse both cords; after: true cord margins anterior ½. 2. No reduction. Female, age 18. Before: 1 x 3 mm; after: 1 x 3 mm. 3. Reduction. Female, age 26. Before: 3.5-4 mm; after: 1 mm. 4. No reduction. Male, age 64. Before: 1 cm³; after: 1 cm³. 5. Elimination of three papilloma, reduction of one. Male, age 35. Before: 3 mm, after: 2 mm. 6. No follow-up. Male, age 66. Before: 1 cm³. 7. No reduction. Male, age 31. Before: 3.5 mm; after: 3 mm. 8. Reduction. Male, age 74. Before: 7-8 mm; after: 5 mm.

From Charts 33 and 34, the following conclusions may be drawn:

1. Of the 25 patients seen, 17 or 68 percent entered therapy.

2. Of the 17 patients entering therapy, 11 or 64.7 percent completed therapy.

3. Of the 11 patients completing therapy, 6 or 54.5 percent had long-term therapy and 5 or 45.5 percent had short-term therapy.

4. Of the 11 patients completing therapy, the results were good, 4 or 36.4 percent; fair, 7 or 63.6 percent.

5. The comparison between males and females seen: males, 14 or 56 percent; females, 11 or 44 percent.

LEUKOPLAKIA AND KERATOSIS

Leukoplakia and keratosis of the vocal folds are premalignant lesions. The etiology remains unknown, but factors which contribute to their onset and development include smoking and vocal misuse and abuse. Many of these patients have a history of vocal abuse. They have competed with environmental noise during their work and/or recreational activities. The cessation of smoking when the individual is a smoker, and/or the elimination of vocal misuse and abuse when such prevails has resulted in a reduction or elimination of the lesions. Patients with these conditions who are nonsmokers and who change their vocal patterns experience a disappearance of the growth(s). Individuals who smoke and who desist from smoking when the condition is made known to them also report a reduction or disappearance of the growth(s). Some individuals continue to smoke but change the vocal pattern and experience a disappearance of the growth(s). Smoking, as has been indicated elsewhere, has a tendency to drop the pitch of the voice to a pitch level which is too low for the individual and therefore creates laryngeal and pharyngeal tensions for the individual.

Surgery has been the main approach in the past. Vocal rehabilitation has not been the usual procedure prior to or following surgery. Some patients seen who have undergone surgical treatment for the removal of these lesions have experienced a return of the growths. As with benign growths, such as nodes, polyps, and contact ulcers, vocal rehabilitation alone or in conjunction with surgery should be considered for leukoplakia and keratosis. Brodnitz (1963) recommends vocal rehabilitation as being helpful for leukoplakia. Peacher (1963) describes vocal therapy as aiding keratosis and leukoplakia. Briess (1957) also finds success in treating leukoplakia by voice therapy. Cracovaner (1965) writes that leukoplakia and hyperkeratotic lesions may be reversed by eliminating causal factors, such as smoking, alcohol, vocal abuse, and chronic infection. What applies to the benign lesions of the vocal folds is even more applicable to the premalignant lesions; the laryngologist uses his discretion as to what procedures will most benefit the patient not only to reduce and eliminate the growth but also to provide information and guidelines which can to some extent remove and eliminate irritants that may be contributing to the condition itself.

Therapy for leukoplakia and keratosis of the vocal folds parallels that of vocal therapy for the benign organic lesions of the folds. Although individuals with leukoplakia and keratosis are usually using a pitch level which is below the optimal pitch, they are not necessarily using a basal or near basal pitch level. The optimal pitch level and range must be located and established at the same time that the balanced oral and nasal resonance is mastered. A vocal image almost invariably exists in these patients.

Few patients experiencing these conditions are afforded vocal rehabilitation; therefore, only a limited number of cases can be reviewed. Charts 35 through 38 describe patients seen with these lesions.

From Charts 35 and 36, the following conclusions may be drawn regarding leukoplakia:

1. Of the 17 patients seen, 9 or 52.9 percent entered therapy.

2. Of the 9 patients entering therapy, 8 or 88.9 percent completed therapy.

3. Of the 8 patients completing therapy, 3 or 37.5 percent had long-term therapy and 5 or 62.5 percent had short-term therapy.

4. Of the 8 patients completing therapy, the results were excellent, 4 or 50 percent; fair, 4 or 50 percent.

5. The comparison between males and females seen: males, 14 or 82.4 percent; females, 3 or 17.6 percent.

From Charts 37 and 38, the following conclusions may be drawn regarding keratosis:

1. Of the 6 patients seen, 5 or 83.3 percent entered therapy.

2. Of the 5 patients entering therapy, 4 or 80 percent completed therapy.

3. Of the 4 patients completing therapy, 2 or 50 percent had long-term therapy and 2 or 50 percent had short-term therapy.

4. Of the 4 patients completing therapy, the results were excellent, 2 or 50 percent; good, 1 or 25 percent; fair, 1 or 25 percent.

5. The comparison between males and females seen: males, 4 or 66.7 percent; females, 2 or 33.3 percent.

PARALYTIC DYSPHONIA

Paralytic dysphonia has been discussed by various authors. Intracordal injection for this condition has been reviewed by Lewy (1966), Toomey and Brown (1967), Boedts, Roels, and Kluyskens (1967), and Rubin (1965a, 1965b, and 1967). Vocal rehabilitation has been presented by Froeschels (1944), Froeschels, Kastein, and Weiss (1955), Weiss (1968) and Cooper (1970a and 1970m). Beginning in 1955, Arnold has written a series of articles covering all aspects of paralytic dysphonia, including description of the paralysis (1962a), vocal rehabilitation (1962b), and intracordal injection (1962c, 1963a). According to Moses (1940), following a thyroidectomy 3 percent of all patients have voice problems which are due to a lesion of the recurrent laryngeal nerve.

Cornut and Pierucci (1968) recommend vocal retraining in paralytic dysphonia regardless of the prognosis, since they feel it always brings either objective or subjective improvement. In regarding the types of therapy, Weiss (1968, p. 383) comments: "In therapy we only ask whether it works. Scientific explanations change anyway with the further development of our basic knowledge, but (therapeutic) factors remain."

The Froeschels approach to this condition, namely that of forceful closure of the vocal folds, is appropriate in the initial stage of therapy when the paralyzed vocal fold is in the paramedian or in the cadaveric position. Weiss (1968, p. 382) agrees:

"The pushing approach in the treatment of cases of the paralysis of the recurrent nerve has proven to have the most important earmark of any therapy: It works."

Whether the paralytic dysphonia is postsurgical, viral, or idiopathic in etiology, a good to excellent prognosis in vocal rehabilitation may be generally forecast for the condition if the paralyzed vocal fold is in the median or paramedian position. Vocal rehabilitation may play a major role in the resolution of the disorder whether the therapy is administered alone or in conjunction with a surgical procedure, such as an injection of Teflon or silicone into the paralyzed vocal fold. Vocal rehabilitation alone is appropriate when the paralyzed vocal cord is in the midline or median position.

When the cord is in the median position, effortful closure of the cord is inappropriate. The median paralysis of the vocal fold does not interfere with the location and identification of the optimal pitch level by the competent voice therapist. The pitch level is almost invariably too low and needs to be raised in order to reach the optimal pitch level. Once the optimal pitch level is located, balanced oral and nasal resonance needs to be sought, if it has not already been established with the location of the optimal pitch level. The supraoptimal pitch level may be used first briefly. When the patient can maintain the supraoptimal pitch level, this pitch level is dropped to the optimal pitch level.

When the paralysis occurs in the paramedian position, the basic approach is, as has been noted, a forceful closure of the cords by emphatic volume starting from the upper range of the voice and extending down to the basal or near basal pitch level. The reverse procedure, from the bottom to the top, may also be used.

The vowels /o/ and /i/ prove extremely effective in effecting closure of the cords with volume. The following therapeutic measures may be considered as an outline.

1. Begin with /o/ prolonging each utterance of the /o/ for a few seconds at the optimal or supraoptimal pitch level. Then proceed to "/o/-one, /o/-two," to ten at the same pitch level.

2. Try the /o/ alone with a staccato utterance at the optimal or supraoptimal pitch level.

3. Alternate between the prolonged /o/ and the staccato /o/ producing one ten times and then the other ten times.

4. Lower the pitch approximately one note and repeat the above exercises.

5. Continue progressing downward one note at a time with the above exercises.

6. When the lowest pitch level has been reached, start with that pitch level and progress upward one note at a time, with the same exercises, until the optimal or supraoptimal pitch is reached.

Once the skips and breaks in the voice as well as the breathiness or hoarseness have been reduced or eliminated, effortful volume should be discontinued for the most part. When the cord is in the cadaveric or intermediate position, a longer period of effortful volume is to be expected. Following the establishment of the optimal pitch level and proper tone focus, if the volume remains too loud, it should be modified at this point.

Depending upon the patient's needs and desires as well as the discretion of the laryngologist, a silicone or Teflon injection may be considered for paralysis in either the paramedian or intermediate position. Some physicians inject Teflon or silicone immediately followed by vocal rehabilitation. Others prefer to try vocal rehabilitation for a period of at least six months. If this program does not prove successful, the physician may elect to inject a synthetic substance into the vocal folds followed by vocal rehabilitation.

Arnold (1962c, p. 363) writes:

> 1. Intrachordal injection should not be considered before all possible attempts at *vocal rehabilitation* by voice therapy have been made. As is well known, many patients are capable of overcoming their vocal disability through systematic development of intralaryngeal compensation and better exploitation of the vocal-auditory feed-back mechanism. . . .*
>
> 2. For the same reason, injection should not be considered *before 6 months have elapsed* since the onset of laryngeal paralysis.*

Regarding the postoperative course, Arnold (p. 367) recom-

---

* *Archives of Otolaryngology,* 76:363, 1962. Copyright 1962, American Medical Association.

mends: "Afterwards, voice therapy should be resumed again for achievement of optimal functional results." Luchsinger and Arnold (1965, p. 174) state:

> Vocal rehabilitation through appropriate *voice therapy* should always be tried first. . . . Following phonosurgical intervention, voice therapy is important to achieve an optimal "tuning" of the artificially changed vocal-cord dimensions.

Rubin (1971, personal communication) injects silicone immediately to afford temporary relief. If cordal function does not return or the paralyzed cord remains in the paramedian or intermediate position, he then injects Teflon. Experience with this modality is generally favorable in experienced hands, according to Rubin.

Some laryngologists do not afford vocal rehabilitation following a synthetic substance injection for paralytic dysphonia. The intracordal injection may well afford a closure of the vocal folds, but the laryngeal control may be irresolute. Immediately after the injection or after a period of some months following the injection, vocal rehabilitation may be necessary for the patient to achieve an efficient voice.

From Charts 39 and 40, the following conclusions may be drawn:

1. Of the 59 patients seen, 29 or 49.2 percent entered therapy.

2. Of the 29 patients entering therapy, 26 or 89.7 percent completed therapy.

3. Of the 26 patients completing therapy, 9 or 34.6 percent had long-term therapy and 17 or 65.4 percent had short-term therapy.

4. Of the 26 patients completing therapy, the results were excellent, 15 or 57.7 percent; good, 6 or 23.1 percent; fair, 5 or 19.2 percent.

5. The comparison between males and females seen: males, 27 or 45.8 percent; females, 32 or 54.2 percent.

PARKINSON'S DISEASE

The voice and speech of the Parkinsonian patient is often markedly impaired. The therapeutic goal for patients with this condition experiencing voice and speech problems is not the goal that might be sought for physiologically normal individuals. Limited goals in voice and speech rehabilitation are appropriate for these patients. The major objective in therapy is that of intelligible speech and adequate voice, not clear speech nor excellent voice.

Greene and Watson (1968) discuss the value of speech amplification for Parkinsonian patients and the need for voice training. Delaini, as cited in Luchsinger and Arnold (1965), reports marked monotomy of voice in six out of ten patients with extrapyramidal disease. Canter (1963) found that normal subjects (control group) used a median fundamental vocal frequency of 106 cycles per second while Parkinsonian patients were at 129 cps. According to this study, Parkinsonian patients are different from the control group in pitch. However, it should be noted that Pronovost (1942), using six superior male speakers, discovered their mean median pitch level to be 132.1 cps, which appears to be comparable to the Parkinsonian patients in Canter's study. Canter found comparable vocal intensity levels and speaking rates for the two groups. Personal clinical experience reveals marked impairment in pitch, tone focus, quality, volume, breath support, and rate in *continuous spontaneous speech.*

Limited as the literature is regarding Parkinson voice and speech, there is an even greater dearth of material relevant to clinical techniques appropriate to vocal and speech rehabilitation of the Parkinsonian patient. Parkinsonian patients require more consideration and attention to their vocal and speech needs.

Patients with Parkinson's disease need a new vocal rate, a new concept of breath control, more expressive lip and tongue movements for greater intelligibility and more oral resonance, a new vocal image, and a new speech image. An increase in volume tends to automatically improve intelligibility and audibility. Unfortunately, the increased volume tends to tire the patient since midsection breathing, which is necessary for the additional volume, is effortful mentally and physically. Nearly all Parkinsonian patients have upper chest breathing.

The increase in volume inclines the patient to a slower rate.

Requesting a patient directly to purposefully slow down the rate, when such a pattern has not been a life style is possibly asking too much. It is possible to indirectly approach the rate by increasing the volume, increasing the articulatory movement, and by coordinating midsection breath support into a spontaneous speaking pattern.

Most patients have too low a pitch range. This vocal habit is clinically explainable because the individual has little breath support and is physically fatigued. Illness of any kind may cause an individual to drop his pitch, often to the basal or near basal pitch range. He utilizes such a pattern because it is easier and more relaxed for him. Unfortunately, the pattern of using this low pitch results in a misused voice that requires effortful volume and lacks flexibility as well as intelligibility.

When the pitch level drops to the basal or near basal pitch level, the tone focus also tends to drop into laryngopharyngeal resonance. Balanced oronasopharyngeal resonance must be established. The tone focus together with the optimal pitch level increases the intelligibility and improves the voice quality. Since the Parkinsonian patient is neurologically handicapped, he may find it laborious to keep his pitch range at the optimal level. Nonetheless, it is possible to do so, even lacking good midsection breath support, if the patient is made aware of the need of using the optimal pitch level.

For those patients who lacked optimal pitch and proper tone focus prior to the onset of the Parkinson's disease, the problem of establishing the correct pitch and tone focus is somewhat more difficult. Although two patients may have a similar severity of the condition, the prognosis for one may be far better than for the second, because the first patient had the proper pitch and tone focus before the condition affected the voice; this patient would be better able to understand and reproduce the pitch level and tone focus.

Frequent tape replays are necessary for the patient to hear and compare the old and new voices and speech patterns. These replays are also essential for the patient to learn to accept the new speech image and the new vocal image.

Though the physiological factor plays an important role in

the patient's willingness and/or ability to cooperate in therapy, the speech and voice images also play a major role in the therapeutic process. The strength of the speech and vocal images, the speech and vocal patterns that have been established because of such images, the length of time which the patient has utilized these speech and voice patterns, the ego strength of the patient, and the role identity to the old patterns as compared to the new patterns all affect the patient's ability to change and to accept the new speech and voice images and thus determine the length of the vocal rehabilitation process and the prognosis of therapy. Vocal psychotherapy is always necessary; psychotherapy may be needed for some patients.

Fourteen patients have been seen with Parkinson's disease. The results appear in Charts 41 and 42.

From Charts 41 and 42, the following conclusions may be drawn:

1. Of the 14 patients seen, 7 or 50 percent entered therapy.

2. Of the 7 patients entering therapy, 4 or 57.1 percent completed therapy.

3. Of the 4 patients completing therapy, 2 or 50 percent had long-term therapy and 2 or 50 percent had short-term therapy.

4. Of the 4 patients completing therapy, the results were good, 1 or 25 percent, and fair, 3 or 75 percent.

5. The comparison between males and females seen: males, 12 or 85.7 percent; females, 2 or 14.3 percent.

6. Results for Parkinsonian patients should be better than indicated here. Most of the patients seen were clinic patients, half of whom elected not to enter therapy. Almost half of those entering therapy did not complete therapy.

OTHER NEUROLOGICAL DISORDERS

These disorders include patients with amyotrophic lateral sclerosis, myasthenia gravis, multiple sclerosis, cerebral palsy, bulbar and pseudobulbar palsy, bulbar poliomyelitis, muscular dystrophy, and dystonia musculorum deformans, among others. Some patients within these various categories have responded better to therapy than other patients; therapy has been more beneficial for some of these neurological disorders than for others. Types of neurological disorders seen which have responded best to therapy are cerebellum tumor (surgically excised) and postcerebral vascular accident dysphonia.

The voice therapist needs to understand that many patients with any of these neurological disorders may not be helped by vocal rehabilitation. Some voice therapy may be used in combination with speech therapy, but voice is not usually a primary concern. If voice therapy is attempted, specific adaptations must be made from the general techniques of vocal rehabilitation to fit the needs and ability of each individual patient.

Perhaps the best approach is speech therapy with some voice therapy and a great deal of supportive therapy. West, Ansberry, and Carr (1957, p. 131) summarize: ". . . but to deny to a group of unfortunate incurables morale-building therapy that should be extended to them is professional malfeasance."

From Charts 43 and 44, the following conclusions may be drawn:

1. Of the 33 patients seen, 11 or 33.3 percent entered therapy.

2. Of the 11 patients entering therapy, 8 or 72.7 percent completed therapy.

3. Of the 8 patients completing therapy, 2 or 25 percent had long-term therapy and 6 or 75 percent had short-term therapy.

4. Of the 8 patients completing therapy, the results were excellent, 1 or 12.5 percent; good, 3 or 37.5 percent; fair, 4 or 50 percent.

5. The comparison between males and females seen: males, 18 or 54.5 percent; females, 15 or 45.5 percent.

6. Patients with severe neurological involvements were seen largely for evaluation only; the results of good were obtained from postcerebral vascular accident dysphonia, brain tumor removal, and multiple sclerosis in the early stages. The excellent result was a spontaneous recovery of neurologically created hypernasality.

PARTIAL CORDECTOMY, COMPLETE CORDECTOMY AND HEMILARYNGECTOMY

Patients who undergo a partial cordectomy, a complete cordectomy, or a hemilaryngectomy should be referred for vocal rehabilitation. According to Pleet (1971, personal communication), a partial or conservative cordectomy involves an excision of a portion of the vocal fold; a complete or radical cordectomy includes the removal of one entire cord with or without the arytenoid cartilage or the vocal process; a hemilaryngectomy involves the removal of an entire half of the larynx, including all of the musculature and usually the thyroid cartilage on one side, may or may not include the arytenoid cartilage, and may include part of the opposite cord anteriorly. The cause of all of those surgical procedures is almost invariably carcinoma of the vocal folds and/or larynx. Irritation whether it be by vocal irritant, such as vocal misuse or abuse, or by smoking should be minimized and where possible, eliminated. Vocal health and vocal ease therefore go together for this type of individual.

Therapy with these dysphonias have afforded encouraging results which warrant further attention and concern by vocal rehabilitationists. A review of patients seen and worked with indicates that, in general, they have experienced pharyngeal and laryngeal tensions due to vocal misuse prior to surgery. The patients have indicated they were hoarse for a long period of time prior to surgery and experienced vocal fatigue during or after brief or prolonged vocal usage.

Approximation of the vocal folds by location and use of the optimal pitch range and moderate volume is most appropriate for a partial cordectomy. The therapy used is similar to that described for paralytic dysphonia when the fold is in the median position. Gentle closure of the vocal folds should be stressed.

For those individuals who have a complete cordectomy or a hemilaryngectomy, therapy has emphasized the location of the most effective pitch level possible with a reasonable closure of the vocal fold against the remaining tissue. The desire and need to use volume is all too apparent to these patients and to their listeners. In the effortful attempt to produce volume, they have the marked tendency to stress the laryngopharyngeal resonance in order to overcome the whisper or the extremely breathy voice which they now have. Vocal hygiene initially is not relevant since competing with noise in cars and talking over television may be helpful in that the additional effort required may assist in closure. Once some closure is occurring, good vocal hygiene must be observed.

Initially, the therapy has stressed the Froeschels approach, that is attempted forceful closure, similar to that for unilateral paralytic dysphonia with the paralyzed fold in the paramedian or in the cadaveric position. The attempted forceful closure occurs only in the early stages of therapy. The optimal pitch level and balanced oronasal resonance must be located as quickly as possible.

As soon as a reasonable tone or pitch level is attained, it is relevant to cease intensive effortful glottal closure and secure a minimum to moderate volume with the optimal pitch level. Vowels such as /o/ and /i/ are useful to afford closure in all stages of therapy. The sound that is produced when closure initially occurs by forceful volume and forceful effort should now be extended to minimum volume and minimum effort from the top of the pitch range extending to the basal and from the basal to the top. A cluster of fairly intelligible sounds or tones centering about the optimal pitch level occurs with some patients. Other patients acquire a clearer tone at the basal or near basal pitch, and still other patients produce a clearer tone at the supraoptimal pitch level. It is appropriate to work within the confines of the patient's vocal ability in that wherever the clearest pitch and tone occurs, so therapy is centered. Ultimately, the optimal pitch level must be located and established for vocal health as well as vocal intelligibility.

The patients experiencing these dysphonias reveal the results shown in Charts 45 and 46.

From Charts 45 and 46, the following conclusions may be drawn:

1. Of the 13 patients seen, 10 or 76.9 percent entered therapy.

2. Of the 10 patients entering therapy, 8 or 80 percent completed therapy.

3. Of the 8 patients completing therapy, 3 or 37.5 percent had long-term therapy and 5 or 62.5 percent had short-term therapy.

4. Of the 8 patients completing therapy, the results were good, 4 or 50 percent; fair, 4 or 50 percent.

5. The comparison between males and females seen: males, 6 or 46.2 percent; females, 7 or 53.8 percent.

ESOPHAGEAL VOICE

This author's goals for esophageal voice training was written for Snidecor (1968, pp. 182-183) and is quoted extensively below:

> The voice of the laryngectomized patient is sadly in need of the vocal rehabilitation efforts we afford the functional and organic voice disorders, such as nodes, polyps, contact ulcer, and myasthenia laryngis. Too often, the patient's demand for speech is abetted by those therapists who have little time, little patience, and little concern for a pleasing, well-modulated quality in the esophageal voice. The aphonic or severe dysphonic whom we see is in no way thought to have terminated therapy because a moderate dysphonia now exists. Rather, we continue our vocal rehabilitation efforts until the voice is clear, easy, and well-modulated. But, for the laryngectomized patient, we have no such goals at the outset of therapy. often we neglect to afford a quality voice, or development of quality in voice for the laryngectomized. It is my view that quality is the essence and not a refinement that should be afforded the laryngectomized patient. Quality should be established at the beginning and not at the conclusion of therapy, since few patients are willing to develop a good voice once they have acquired some form of esophageal voice. We should not rush the patient into voice, but into an understanding of how to produce an efficient and well-modulated voice at the outset of therapy. It may slow down therapy at the beginning, and frustrate the patient not to speak earlier or faster, but the final result is much better and a goal to be sought, if excellence is sought.

The combined emotional, psychological, and physical trauma created by a surgical procedure resulting in a laryngectomy is continued with the realization of esophageal voice and its use. It has been estimated that 30 percent of all laryngectomized patients never learn esophageal voice. Usually, but perhaps erroneously, the patient is faulted for not developing esophageal voice, let alone good esophageal voice.

In this author's experience the failure to develop esophageal voice is essentially psychological, not physiological. Some patients who have experienced extensive surgical and medical procedures, including cobalt treatment, have been able to speak again with excellent voices. Carrell (1963) does not believe that the surgical variables affect the success of esophageal voice training. He (p. 258) says:

We have come to believe that the single most important and overriding consideration for successful rehabilitation lies in the area of the psychological reaction of the patient. It follows from this that the primary problem is one of psychotherapy in the broader sense, and the training is structured in this way. The greatest emphasis is placed on an effort to understand the patient's total problem and his feelings.

The will to speak is the key, and that key must often be turned in the right direction for each patient.

The vocal image is one of those keys that unlock the patient's desire, will, and ability to speak again effectively. The vocal image extensively prevails among laryngectomized patients. The laryngectomized patient is concerned with how he will sound. He compares the new sound or voice to the presurgical voice, judging that new sound for its ease, flexibility, durability, and aesthetic listenability. He is also concerned with how other people will accept the new sound.

There are three categories of esophageal speakers. The first group attempts to develop esophageal voice but fails to do so. The second group develops inept esophageal voice which is difficult to understand and thus trying for the listener as well as for the speaker. The third group develops very effective esophageal voice.

Some of the reasons for the first two groups are as follows:

1. In the first group, the patient may feel that it is not worth the effort to learn to speak again. He himself is not adequately motivated to speak. He may be sufficiently accepted by himself or by his group to remain silent. Seldom is he physically unable to practice at developing the new sound. In the few cases where the patient is physically fatigued, therapy must proceed slowly. In the second group, the patient may not be motivated to learn to speak fluently. He is internally adjusted to and externally accepted by society to speak mostly in either monosyllabic or phrase responses. When fully articulated sentences are attempted, intelligibility, which may already be impaired, is further affected. In both groups, the patient may be emotionally and psychologically unprepared and unwilling to take the time and the effort to develop a new voice. The new sound does not appeal to him, or to his wife, or to someone important or influential in

his life; therefore, he makes little or a limited attempt to achieve the new voice.

2. The therapist is either unaware of or unable to meet the particular and specific needs of the patient. For example, if the patient has had cobalt treatment, he may be unable to produce an easy or clear basic belch sound consistently; the therapist should not expect an easy, consistent sound production, and the patient should understand why this sound production is difficult. The therapist may fail to explore and discuss the vocal image and determine how the patient feels about the esophageal voice and his acceptance of it.

3. Laryngectomees as teachers are an unknown quality per se. Laryngectomized individuals who teach esophageal voice may attempt to superimpose their specific technique of esophageal voice training upon the patient who may need a greater number of approaches instead of one specific method. In most instances, these laryngectomees are not professionally trained and are usually qualified only in that they themselves are laryngectomized and have learned to speak again using esophageal voice. Such a situation is analogous to one who has experienced an articulation or stuttering or voice problem, and having overcome it, becomes automatically qualified to direct others to surmount their respective speech or voice disorder. The lack of a quality voice or an efficient esophageal voice often results because the therapist is not professionally trained to isolate, identify, and establish an excellent, basic belch sound or voice initially in the patient. In vocal rehabilitation with patients who are not laryngectomized, it is essential to develop the optimal pitch level, proper tone focus, flexibility of tone, and midsection breath support. The same is true of esophageal voice. Unless the therapist is prepared to fully develop the patient's esophageal voice to its potential, he should not be teaching esophageal voice.

Esophageal Voice Training

The following are necessary steps in the esophageal voice training:

1. It is important that the therapist be able to produce good esophageal voice himself and demonstrate this voice for the pa-

tient. The therapist should serve as a model for the patient and should be able to demonstrate each step and instruction as he directs the patient.

2. The therapist seeks to find the easiest and best method for the patient to produce a basic belch sound. The patient is directed to open his mouth slightly and inhale a small amount of air. For those who cannot inhale the air, they are told to swallow the air, that is forcing the air into the esophagus using the tongue and pharyngeal muscles. The method developed by Doehler (1956) is used: open mouth, close mouth, swallow air, open mouth and return air. Patients may initially learn to produce the basic belch sound by the swallow method and then move to the inhalation approach, or begin and master the sound using the inhalation method exclusively. Some patients are helped by carbonated drinks at first. Of all the laryngectomized patients seen, only one or two have been unable to produce the basic and essential belch sound. Nearly all patients can produce and control the isolated belch.

3. In producing the basic belch sound, the patient usually finds it easiest to produce an /i/, /a/, and /o/. If the patient is unable to produce these vowels in isolation after a reasonable period of practice, a plosive consonant, such as /b/, is added so that the patient practices "be," "ba," and "bo." The patient needs to practice the /i/, /a/, and /o/ until he can produce the sound at will consistently and automatically. At this point, the patient obtains some mastery of the sound by producing the sound in a staccato fashion and by prolonging the sound. The quality of the sound must be clear, firm, and full. As soon as these three sounds are clearly produced, the patient practices and masters the production of the other vowels and diphthongs.

4. Following the practice of these sounds, the patient adds a consonant to the beginning of each vowel and diphthong. The consonants commonly used are /b/, /p/, /t/, /d/, /k/, and /g/, the plosive sounds.

5 and 6. At this point, the patient may either be directed to add final consonant sounds to the initial consonant and vowel or diphthong or he may be instructed to practice the other initial consonant sounds in combination with the vowels and diph-

thongs. The therapist and patient determine which is easier and more appropriate for the patient. Both of these aspects of training must be mastered before continuing to the next step.

7. Following the production of all initial and final consonant sounds, including blends, with all vowels and diphthongs, the patient progresses to two- and three-word phrases.

8. When the patient is able to produce two and three words in combination efficiently and automatically, he is instructed to practice with inflectional and intonational patterns so that a normal and natural rhythm is established for the esophageal voice. Following the mastery of two- or three-word phrases, he proceeds to longer utterances.

9. The patient must learn to gauge his ability to control the sound and his breath supply so that the word at the end of the sentence is as clear as the beginning of the sentence. The patient also practices taking in air between phrases in longer sentences.

10. The patient practices spontaneous speech. For those who feel uncomfortable producing spontaneous words, phrases, and sentences in any of the above steps, they may read aloud from word lists, books, and newspapers, depending upon their ability and inclination.

The essence of an excellent esophageal voice is the development of a basic, clear, controlled, and automatic single vowel or diphthong. The mastery of step 3 is essentially the mastery of esophageal voice. If the tone is not clear or automatic at this point, everything else will fail. The voice or speech pattern that relies upon a gurgly or unclear tone with poor or inept control will have initial acceptance, but once the "honeymoon" period (from six months to a year or so) is over, listener acceptability will decline and eventually result in speaker disinclination. The cycle becomes vicious with the extent and degree of speech deterioration. The patient will not be willing to go back and master a good tone after completing all of the steps; therefore, he must master the tone first. Regarding therapy, Peacher (1963, p. 3107) suggests: "The part [section] on optimum pitch and pitch range with work on melody and a resonant quality enables those with esophageal voices to develop more pleasing tones."

Optimal pitch and balanced oronasopharyngeal tone focus for

the esophageal voice are seldom discussed concepts and apparently even less sought after goals in the development of the esophageal voice. The esophageal voice has within it an optimal pitch level and range as does the normal speaking voice. With the development of the potential optimal pitch and proper tone focus, there is greater intelligibility, greater carrying power, and greater naturalness to the voice. The use of the optimal pitch also eliminates some of the low grating sound caused by the use of the basal or near basal pitch.

Articulation is a minor concern in the procurement of a new speaking voice. It is the voice itself which must be redefined and reaffirmed, not the articulation. Therefore, practice on mastery of the voice, of the basic sound until it is easily produced and controlled will enable the patient to use his normal articulatory process. The esophageal speaker may emphasize tongue and lip movements to obtain more intelligible speech.

Several problems must be avoided or overcome in learning the esophageal voice. One is the gurgly or wet voice which is caused by phlegm. Some patients produce more phlegm than others, and anxiety contributes to a greater flow of phlegm. The patient must be assured that this condition is temporary, since it is related to anxieties and fears of the speaker in the production of the new voice. The patient is directed to swallow this phlegm as often as necessary so that the esophageal lips are clear.

Another problem to be avoided is the audible intake of air, which produces a click or gulp sound. This is caused by tenseness and by taking too much air in at one time. The patient is directed to take in small amounts of air more frequently while he is learning esophageal voice.

The patient must be warned that learning esophageal voice is fatiguing mentally and physically. The muscles of the midsection and of the throat become fatigued due to the new stresses and pressures upon them. The patient must realize that this is a temporary condition. The patient must also be counseled about facial grimaces. These may occur as the patient attempts to learn control of the basic sound.

The patient must be warned that he may have a morning

voice that occurs with normal speakers as well. The morning voice is at the lowest pitch level because the neck musculature as well as the entire body musculature is lax. This voice is difficult to produce. The patient must practice from fifteen to thirty minutes to clear up the condition.

Midsection breath support is of concern only when the basic sound is controlled and automatic. Support of the basic sound through midsection breathing is then stressed. The volume of the esophageal voice will increase with the use of midsection breath support. The same techniques for increasing volume and controlling breath support for normal speakers is also applicable for esophageal speakers.

Coughing may occur if the esophageal speaker forces his voice in volume, in rate, or in pitch. He must also be aware that the voice will tire at first; he will be able to speak for longer periods of time as he practices and progresses until eventually he will be able to speak comfortably for long periods of time. Taking in too much air can create hiccoughs, flatulence, and midsection pain. The patient must learn through experimentation the amount of air intake needed to produce a fluid, comfortable voice and speech pattern.

Rate of speech is important in the esophageal voice. Too fast a speaking rate and the articulation falters. If the rate is too slow, the listener may not be receptive and the patient loses confidence in himself and in his speech. Within the first year or so, the patient will be accepted with his impaired rate of speech. This transition period is the time for practice and for mastery of esophageal voice. The speech rate will develop as the mastery of the sound develops. With the automaticity of sound production which is clear, the individual can move on to a faster rate. If the patient rushes into a fast rate too quickly to please himself or his listener, he may develop a poor speech pattern which lacks intelligibility and listenability and which is not acceptable to himself or to others.

Unfortunately, as the patient progresses in the mastery of esophageal voice, he all too frequently has the tendency to emulate his own old speech rate, which was much faster than the one he can now control, or he may emulate the speech rate of those around him, which again is too rapid for esophageal speech at this time. One method of slowing down this type of speaker is to play back his speech on a tape machine. He quickly realizes he is difficult to understand, since he himself may have to strain to follow what he has just recorded. Gulping and grimacing may develop from an attempt at speech too rapid for this current speech ability. Eventually, the esophageal speaker must develop a speech pattern which is comfortable for him and which is highly listenable.

The laryngectomized patient without a voice has a tendency to be anxious. It is essential to develop the speaking voice as quickly as possible without inept habits. Intensive therapy, two to five sessions per week, is recommended for the first month or so. After this the therapist can decrease the frequency of therapy and afford the patient more responsibility for his vocal rehabilitation.

In the beginning of therapy, a laryngectomized patient with good esophageal voice and speech should be brought into the therapy session with the new patient who is attempting to learn esophageal voice and speech. The accomplished esophageal speaker serves as a model and a motivating force for the new patient. For some patients, tape recordings of good esophageal speakers may be used.

If the laryngectomized individual wishes, he may secure a mechanical instrument which will afford him some form of intelligible communication during the process of learning esophageal voice or in addition to his esophageal voice. Most patients are willing to try to master esophageal voice without the assistance of a mechanical instrument during this training process. Of course, an instrument may be necessary for the individual who is simply unable to learn esophageal voice.

VOCAL IMAGE

The factors that may influence the learning of esophageal voice, or the mastery of this voice, are mixed factors. One of the most prominent factors among those patients who drop out or those who continue but do not produce good or excellent voice is the concern of the vocal image. A vocal image exists within all speakers in that they visualize themselves as being a certain type of speaker with a certain type of voice.

Patients, especially women, who enter vocal rehabilitation without a larynx and seek a new voice are up against not only an internal vocal image, a sound, a voice they knew and accepted, but also a vocal image of society that the voice should sound a given way and that variation from it attracts and offends.

Society dictates an acceptable vocal image. The extremely low-pitched esophageal voice is noticed immediately and reacted to sharply. Its sound and production are so different for the listener who is essentially unprepared for this sound that its very existence tends to interfere with communication. If Van Riper's (1963, p. 16) criteria of a speech defect is applied *"Speech is defective when it deviates so far from the speech of other people that it calls attention to itself, interferes with communication or causes its possessor to be maladjusted,"* then an esophageal voice is often a speech or voice defect. As therapists training individuals in esophageal voice, it is incumbent upon us that we initiate a program of public education to be carried out by national and state speech therapy associations through the mass media. The need to alert and to train society to accept the esophageal voice is obligatory and imperative. At present, what we are doing is teaching individuals to use a voice that is not readily acceptable to society or to themselves.

Laryngectomized patients not only have vocal images that are related to their life style and role identity, but also have extremely strong vocal images regarding the new voice, its sound, its fluency, its durability, and its acceptance by society. The immediate or abrupt change in vocal identity due to the surgical procedure creates intensive and extensive changes in regard to one's voice. The laryngectomized patient continues vocal therapy because he wants to communicate. But all the while he is not internally pleased with the tone or the production of his new voice. Therefore, he may not fully or extensively practice the new voice.

The vocal image the patient had prior to the laryngectomy

---

* Charles Van Riper, *Speech Correction: Principles and Methods,* 4th ed., p. 16. Copyright 1963, Prentice-Hall, Englewood Cliffs, New Jersey.

may influence the acquisition of the esophageal voice. The individual who was successful as a conversational speaker using a normal voice has been found to be negative toward the new sound of the esophageal voice and the new vocal image. Initially, a number of patients in this category have not been cooperative for a period of one to three months. These patients must be assured and convinced that the slow halting speech pattern is temporary and that they will be able to develop good speech styles somewhat commensurate to their former speech presentation.

Training the esophageal speaker is more than just training a speaker to use a new voice. It is acclimating the laryngectomee to a new sound, a new method of voice, a new vocal identity and a vocal image. During therapy, patients will experience and exhibit many negative feelings, such as hostility, aggression, despair, anger, frustration, hopelessness, and withdrawal. The therapist must be able to understand and to cope with all of these normal feelings. The patient must be guided into developing a voice that is easily intelligible, comfortable, and listenable and that will allow the patient to be himself and to be acceptable as a person and as a speaker.

Vocal psychotherapy is an inherent aspect of vocal rehabilitation and with esophageal voice, vocal psychotherapy is greater in need and extent, as it involves the laryngectomized patient more extensively and more fully. Extended vocal psychotherapy is often apropos. The patient should be aware of and understand his own feelings and reaction to this type of voice. He should also be prepared for the reactions of others and understand the effect this voice has on listeners. The patient may need to be counseled that even his worst efforts initially will be accepted by society for a relatively short period of time, perhaps six to twelve months. But if these early efforts are not improved and refined so that the voice becomes smooth and flexible, communication may be severely impaired both for the speaker and the listener. If vocal psychotherapy is not sufficient to help or assist the patient in accepting and using the esophageal voice, psychotherapy then becomes an essential and integral aspect of the retraining program.

The entire point and purpose of vocal rehabilitation for the laryngectomized speaker is to teach him esophageal voice and to make him feel natural and normal with a voice that is different. As one laryngectomized patient said, "Good esophageal voice is making me feel and be normal."

From Charts 47 and 48, the following conclusions may be drawn:

1. Of the 55 patients seen, 40 or 72.7 percent entered therapy.

2. Of the 40 patients entering therapy, 30 or 75 percent completed therapy.

3. Of the 30 patients completing therapy, 4 or 13.3 percent had long-term therapy and 26 or 86.7 percent had short-term therapy.

4. Of the 30 patients completing therapy, the results were excellent, 15 or 50 percent; good, 8 or 26.7 percent; fair, 7 or 23.3 percent.

5. The comparison between males and females seen: males, 48 or 87.3 percent; females, 7 or 12.7 percent.

INDEX OF CHARTS WHICH FOLLOW

CHART 1—FUNCTIONAL MISPHONIA (486)

Columns under **Therapy** are grouped as Long-term (Excel., Good, Fair) and Short-term (Excel., Good, Fair).

Age	Patients Seen M	F	Evaluation Only M	F	Entered Therapy M	F	Incon-clusive M	F	Completed Therapy M	F	Long-term Excel. M	F	Long-term Good M	F	Long-term Fair M	F	Short-term Excel. M	F	Short-term Good M	F	Short-term Fair M	F
0-10	5	5	4	1	1	4	1			4		1						1	2	2		1
11-20	19	15	5	5	14	10		1	14	9	2	3					9	5	8	3	3	
21-30	40	48	10	16	30	32	3	8	30	32	9	5	1	1			20	19	7	3		7
31-40	68	41	8	11	60	30	3	4	57	22	10	4		2	1		36	10	1	4	3	2
41-50	76	56	24	14	52	42	3	3	49	38	5	2					33	23	1	6	4	3
51-60	24	50	8	22	16	28		1	13	25		4					6	17	3	5	1	1
61-70	8	21	3	10	5	11			5	10							2	5		3		1
71+	4	6	3	1	1	5			1	5			1					2				
Subtotal	244	242	65	80	179	162	11	17	168	145	26	19	2	3	1		106	82	22	26	11	15
Total	486		145		341		28		313		45		5		1		188		48		26	

CHART 2—FUNCTIONAL MISPHONIA (486)

	Patients Seen			Evaluation Only	Entered Therapy	Inconclusive	Completed Therapy	Therapy					
									Long-term			Short-term	
	M	F	Total				Excel.	Good	Fair	Excel.	Good	Fair
Totals	244	242	486	145	341	28	313	45	5	1	188	48	26
Percentage	50.2	49.8		29.8	70.2	8.2	91.8	14.4	1.6	.3	60.1	15.3	8.3

Therapy Length Totals		Therapy Results Totals		
Long-term	Short-term	Excel.	Good	Fair
Totals 51	262	233	53	27
Percentage 16.3	83.7	74.4	16.9	8.6

CHART 3—FALSETTO (34)

Age	Patients Seen		Evaluation Only		Entered Therapy		Incon-clusive		Completed Therapy		Long-term Excel.		Long-term Good		Long-term Fair		Short-term Excel.		Short-term Good		Short-term Fair	
	M	F	M	F	M	F	M	F	M	F	M	F	M	F	M	F	M	F	M	F	M	F
0-10																						
11-20	17	1	5		12		2		10		1		1		1		6		1			
21-30	11		3		8				8		2						4				2	
31-40	1				1				1								1					
41-50	1	2		2	1				1								1					
51-60																						
61-70		1		1		1																
71+																						
Subtotal	30	4	8	4	22		2		20		3		1		1		12		1		2	
Total	34		12		22		2		20		3		1		1		12		1		2	

CHART 4—FALSETTO (34)

| | Patients Seen | | | Evaluation Only | Entered Therapy | Inconclusive | Completed Therapy | Therapy | | | | | |
	M	F	Total					Excel.	Long-term Good	Fair	Excel.	Short-term Good	Fair
Totals	30	4	34	12	22	2	20	3	1	1	12	1	2
Percentage	88.2	11.8		35.3	64.7	9.1	90.9	15	5	5	60	5	10

| | Therapy Length Totals | | Therapy Results Totals | | |
	Long-term	Short-term	Excel.	Good	Fair
Totals	5	15	15	2	3
Percentage	25	75	75	10	15

CHART 5—VENTRICULAR PHONATION (11)

Age	Patients Seen		Evaluation Only		Entered Therapy		Incon-clusive		Completed Therapy		Excel.		Long-term Good		Fair		Excel.		Short-term Good		Fair	
													Therapy									
	M	F	M	F	M	F	M	F	M	F	M	F	M	F	M	F	M	F	M	F	M	F
0-10																							
11-20																							
21-30	1				1		1																
31-40	2	2	1		1	2		2	1		1												
41-50		3		2		1				1										1			
51-60	1		1																				
61-70																							
71+		2		1		1				1								1					
Subtotal	4	7	2	3	2	4	1	2	1	2	1							1		1			
Total	11		5		6		3		3		1							1		1			

(Long-term
Inconclusive)

CHART 6—VENTRICULAR PHONATION (11)

| | Patients Seen | | | Evalu-ation Only | Entered Therapy | Incon-clusive | Com-pleted Therapy | Therapy | | | | | |
| | | | | | | | | Long-term | | | Short-term | | |
	M	F	Total				Excel.	Excel.	Good	Fair	Excel.	Good	Fair
Totals	4	7	11	5	6	3	3	1			1	1	
Percentage	36.4	63.6		45.5	54.5	50	50	33.3			33.3	33.3	

| | Therapy Length Totals | | Therapy Results Totals | | |
	Long-term	Short-term	Excel.	Good	Fair
Totals	1	2	2	1	
Percentage	33.3	66.7	66.7	33.3	

CHART 7—HYSTERICAL APHONIA (9)

Age	Patients Seen M	F	Evaluation Only M	F	Entered Therapy M	F	Incon-clusive M	F	Completed Therapy M	F	Therapy Long-term Excel. M	F	Long-term Good M	F	Fair M	F	Short-term Excel. M	F	Short-term Good M	F	Fair M	F
0-10																						
11-20																						
21-30		2		1		1		1														
31-40		2		1		1				1										1		
41-50		2		2																		
51-60		1				1				1		1										
61-70		1				1				1		1										
71+	1				1				1		1											
Subtotal	1	8		4	1	4		1	1	3	1	2								1		
Total	9		4		5		1		4		3								1			

CHART 8—HYSTERICAL APHONIA (9)

	Patients Seen			Evaluation Only	Entered Therapy	Inconclusive	Completed Therapy	Therapy				
									Long-term		Short-term	
	M	F	Total				Excel.	Excel.	Good	Fair	Good	Fair
Totals	1	8	9	4	5	1	4	3			1	
Percentage	11.1	88.9		44.4	55.6	20	80	75			25	

	Therapy Length Totals		Therapy Results Totals		
	Long-term	Short-term	Excel.	Good	Fair
Totals		4	3	1	
Percentage		100	75	25	

CHART 9—HYSTERICAL DYSPHONIA (9)

Age	Patients Seen		Evaluation Only		Entered Therapy		Incon-clusive		Completed Therapy		Therapy											
											Excel.		Long-term Good		Fair		Excel.		Short-term Good		Fair	
	M	F	M	F	M	F	M	F	M	F	M	F	M	F	M	F	M	F	M	F	M	F
0-10																						
11-20																						
21-30		1				1				1											1	
31-40	2	2			2	2			2	2	1						1	1		1		
41-50		2		2																		
51-60		2		1		1				1								1				
61-70																						
71+																						
Subtotal	2	7		3	2	4			2	4	1						1	2		2		
Total	9		3		6				6		1						3		2			

CHART 10—HYSTERICAL DYSPHONIA (9)

| | Patients Seen | | | Evaluation Only | Entered Therapy | Inconclusive | Completed Therapy | Therapy | | | | | |
| | | | | | | | | Long-term | | | Short-term | | |
	M	F	Total				Excel.	Excel.	Good	Fair	Excel.	Good	Fair
Totals	2	7	9	3	6		6	1			3	2	
Percentage	22.2	77.8		33.3	66.7		100	16.7			50	33.3	

| | Therapy Length Totals | | Therapy Results Totals | | |
	Long-term	Short-term	Excel.	Good	Fair
Totals	1	5	4	2	
Percentage	16.7	83.3	66.7	33.3	

CHART 11—FUNCTIONAL APHONIA (5)

Age	Patients Seen M	F	Evaluation Only M	F	Entered Therapy M	F	Inconclusive M	F	Completed Therapy M	F	Long-term Excel. M	F	Long-term Good M	F	Fair M	F	Short-term Excel. M	F	Short-term Good M	F	Fair M	F
0-10																						
11-20		1				1				1								1				
21-30																						
31-40	1				1				1								1					
41-50		1				1				1								1				
51-60																						
61-70		2				2				2								2				
71+																						
Subtotal	1	4			1	4			1	4							1	4				
Total	5				5				5								5					

CHART 12—FUNCTIONAL APHONIA (5)

	Patients Seen			Evalu- ation Only	Entered Therapy	Incon- clusive	Com- pleted Therapy	Therapy					
									Long-term		Short-term		
	M	F	Total					Excel.	Good	Fair	Excel.	Good	Fair
Totals	1	4	5		5		5				5		
Percentage	20	80			100		100				100		

Therapy Length Totals		Therapy Results Totals		
Long-term	Short-term	Excel.	Good	Fair
Totals	5	5		
Percentage	100	100		

CHART 13—SPASTIC DYSPHONIA (42)

Age	Patients Seen M	Patients Seen F	Evaluation Only M	Evaluation Only F	Entered Therapy M	Entered Therapy F	Incon-clusive M	Incon-clusive F	Completed Therapy M	Completed Therapy F	Long-term Excel. M	Long-term Excel. F	Long-term Good M	Long-term Good F	Long-term Fair M	Long-term Fair F	Short-term Excel. M	Short-term Excel. F	Short-term Good M	Short-term Good F	Short-term Fair M	Short-term Fair F
0-10																						
11-20	1	1		1	1		1															
21-30	3		1		2		2															
31-40	6	11	3	6	3	5	1	5	2		1		1									
41-50	7	6	3	3	4	3	3	3	1				1									
51-60		3		1		2		1		1				1								
61-70		1				1				1						1						
71+	1	2	1	1		1				1						1						
Subtotal	18	24	8	12	10	12	7	9	3	3	1		2	1		2						
Total	42		20		22		16		6		1		3		2							

(4 Long-term Inconclusive)

CHART 14—SPASTIC DYSPHONIA (42)

	Patients Seen			Evaluation Only	Entered Therapy	Inconclusive Therapy	Completed Therapy	Therapy Excel.	Therapy Long-term Good	Fair	Short-term Good	Fair
	M	F	Total									
Totals	18	24	42	20	22	16	6	1	3	2		
Percentage	42.9	57.1		47.6	52.4	72.7	27.3	16.7	50	33.3		

	Therapy Length Totals		Therapy Results Totals		
	Long-term	Short-term	Excel.	Good	Fair
Totals	6		1	3	2
Percentage	100		16.7	50	33.3

CHART 15—INCIPIENT SPASTIC DYSPHONIA (21)

Age	Patients Seen M	F	Evaluation Only M	F	Entered Therapy M	F	Incon-clusive M	F	Completed Therapy M	F	Long-term Excel. M	F	Long-term Good M	F	Long-term Fair M	F	Short-term Excel. M	F	Short-term Good M	F	Short-term Fair M	F
0-10																						
11-20																						
21-30		2				2		2														
31-40	4	4	1	2	3	2	1		2	2	1	1							1	1		
41-50		2		1		1				2								1				
51-60	2	3	1	1	1	2	1			2						1		1				
61-70		3		2		1				1								1				
71+	1				1				1								1					
Subtotal	7	14	2	6	5	8	2	2	3	6	1	1				1	1	3	1	1		
Total	21		8		13		4		9		2				1		4		2			

(*Therapy* groups the outcome columns: *Long-term* and *Short-term*, each with *Excel.*, *Good*, *Fair*.)

CHART 16—INCIPIENT SPASTIC DYSPHONIA (21)

	Patients Seen			Evaluation Only	Entered Therapy	Inconclusive	Completed Therapy	Therapy					
								Long-term			Short-term		
	M	F	Total					Excel.	Good	Fair	Excel.	Good	Fair
Totals	7	14	21	8	13	4	9	2		1	4	2	
Percentage	33.3	66.7		38.1	61.9	30.8	69.2	22.2		11.1	44.4	22.2	

	Therapy Length Totals		Therapy Results Totals		
	Long-term	Short-term	Excel.	Good	Fair
Totals	3	6	6	2	1
Percentage	33.3	66.7	66.7	22.2	11.1

CHART 17—NASALITY—FUNCTIONAL (44)

Age	Patients Seen M	F	Evaluation Only M	F	Entered Therapy M	F	Incon-clusive M	F	Completed Therapy M	F	Excel. M	F	Long-term Good M	F	Fair M	F	Therapy Excel. M	F	Short-term Good M	F	Fair M	F
0-10	10	6	6	4	4	2			4	2	2			1			1		1	1		
11-20	9	8	5	1	4	7		1	4	6	2	2		1	1			2	1	1		
21-30	1	3		2	1	1		1	1		1											
31-40	1		1																			
41-50	2	3		3	2		1		1										1			
51-60		1		1																		
61-70																						
71+																						
Subtotal	23	21	12	11	11	10	1	2	10	8	5	2		2	1		1	2	3	2		
Total	44		23		21		3		18		7		2		1		3		5			

CHART 18—NASALITY—FUNCTIONAL (44)

	Patients Seen			Evaluation Only	Entered Therapy	Inconclusive	Completed Therapy	Therapy					
	M	F	Total					Long-term			Short-term		
								Excel.	Good	Fair	Excel.	Good	Fair
Totals	23	21	44	23	21	3	18	7	2	1	3	5	
Percentage	52.3	47.7		52.3	47.7	14.3	85.7	38.9	11.1	5.6	16.7	27.8	

	Therapy Length Totals		Therapy Results Totals		
	Long-term	Short-term	Excel.	Good	Fair
Totals	10	8	10	7	1
Percentage	55.6	44.4	55.6	38.9	5.6

CHART 19—NASALITY—ORGANIC (11)

	Patients Seen		Evaluation Only		Entered Therapy		Incon-clusive		Completed Therapy		Therapy Long-term Excel.		Long-term Good		Fair		Short-term Excel.		Short-term Good		Fair	
Age	M	F	M	F	M	F	M	F	M	F	M	F	M	F	M	F	M	F	M	F	M	F
0-10	2	3	1	1	1	2			1	2		1	1					1				
11-20	1	3	1			3				3		1				1				1		
21-30	1				1				1				1									
31-40																						
41-50	1		1																			
51-60																						
61-70																						
71+																						
Subtotal	5	6	3	1	2	5			2	5		2	2			1		1		1		
Total	11		4		7				7		2		2		1		1		1			

CHART 20—NASALITY—ORGANIC (11)

	Patients Seen			Evaluation Only	Entered Therapy	Inconclusive	Completed Therapy	Therapy Long-term			Therapy Short-term		
	M	F	Total					Excel.	Good	Fair	Excel.	Good	Fair
Totals	5	6	11	4	7		7	2	2	1	1	1	
Percentage	45.5	54.5		36.4	63.6		100	28.6	28.6	14.3	14.3	14.3	

	Therapy Length Totals Long-term	Short-term	Therapy Results Totals Excel.	Good	Fair
Totals	5	2	3	3	1
Percentage	71.4	28.6	42.8	42.8	14.3

CHART 21—BOWED VOCAL FOLDS—FUNCTIONAL (32)

Age	Patients Seen M	F	Evaluation Only M	F	Entered Therapy M	F	Incon-clusive M	F	Completed Therapy M	F	Long-term Excel. M	F	Long-term Good M	F	Long-term Fair M	F	Short-term Excel. M	F	Short-term Good M	F	Short-term Fair M	F
0-10	1				1		1															
11-20	1				1				1								1					
21-30	5	3	1		4	3		1	4	2	1						3	1		1		
31-40	1	2			1	2			1	2								1			1	1
41-50	8	2		1	8	1			8	1	3	1					5					
51-60	2	4	1	2	1	2			1	2	1	1						1				
61-70	2		1		1				1										1			
71+		1				1				1								1				
Subtotal	20	12	3	3	17	9	1	1	16	8	5	2					9	4	1	1	1	1
Total	32		6		26		2		24		7						13		2		2	

CHART 22—BOWED VOCAL FOLDS—FUNCTIONAL (32)

	Patients Seen			Evaluation Only	Entered Therapy	Inconclusive	Completed Therapy	Therapy					
								Long-term			Short-term		
	M	F	Total					Excel.	Good	Fair	Excel.	Good	Fair
Totals	20	12	32	6	26	2	24	7			13	2	2
Percentage	62.5	37.5		18.75	81.25	7.7	92.3	29.2			54.2	8.3	8.3

	Therapy Length Totals		Therapy Results Totals		
	Long-term	Short-term	Excel.	Good	Fair
Totals	7	17	20	2	2
Percentage	29.2	70.8	83.3	8.3	8.3

CHART 23—BOWED VOCAL FOLDS—ORGANIC (10)*

Age	Patients Seen M	F	Evaluation Only M	F	Entered Therapy M	F	Incon-clusive M	F	Completed Therapy M	F	Long-term Excel. M	F	Long-term Good M	F	Long-term Fair M	F	Short-term Excel. M	F	Short-term Good M	F	Short-term Fair M	F
0-10																						
11-20		1				1				1		1										
21-30	1	2			1	2	1	2														
31-40		1				1				1		1										
41-50	1				1				1				1									
51-60	1	2			1	2			1	2							1	1		1		
61-70																		1				
71+	1					1				1												
Subtotal	3	7			3	7	1	2	2	5		2	1				1	2		1		
Total	10		10		10		3		7		2		1				3		1			

Therapy results are grouped as Long-term (Excel., Good, Fair) and Short-term (Excel., Good, Fair).

* Nodules—7 (5 no surgery; 2 postoperative); Polyps—1 (postoperative); Polypoid degeneration—2 (1 no surgery; 1 postoperative)

CHART 24—BOWED VOCAL FOLDS—ORGANIC (10)*

	Patients Seen			Evaluation Only	Entered Therapy	Inconclusive Therapy	Completed Therapy	Therapy					
								Long-term			Short-term		
	M	F	Total					Excel.	Good	Fair	Excel.	Good	Fair
Totals	3	7	10		10	3	7	2	1		3	1	
Percentage	30	70			100	30	70	28.6	14.3		42.9	14.3	

	Therapy Length Totals		Therapy Results Totals		
	Long-term	Short-term	Excel.	Good	Fair
Totals	3	4	5	2	
Percentage	42.9	57.1	71.4	28.6	

* Nodules—7 (5 no surgery; 2 postoperative); Polyps—1 (postoperative); Polypoid degeneration—2 (1 no surgery; 1 postoperative)

CHART 25—NODULES (254)

The Long-term and Short-term outcome groups fall under the heading "Therapy".

Age	Patients Seen		Evaluation Only		Entered Therapy		Inconclusive		Completed Therapy		Long-term Excel.		Long-term Good		Long-term Fair		Short-term Excel.		Short-term Good		Short-term Fair	
	M	F	M	F	M	F	M	F	M	F	M	F	M	F	M	F	M	F	M	F	M	F
0-10	11	4	4	4	7				7		1		2				5		1			
11-20	9	8	2	3	7	5	1		6	5	2	3					1	2	1	6		1
21-30	13	34	4	7	9	27		2	9	25	2	8					4	10	1	2	2	2
31-40	27	33	3	10	24	23		1	24	22	4	6					13	12	5	1	2	3
41-50	29	31	10	5	19	26	2	3	17	23	4	6	1			1	5	12	3	3	4	5
51-60	10	27		6	10	21	1		9	21	2	3	2				4	10			1	2
61-70	6	8	1	4	5	4	1	1	4	3							4	1		1		
71+	2	2	1		1	2			1	2					1			1				
Subtotal	107	147	25	39	82	108	5	7	77	101	15	26	5		1	1	36	48	11	13	9	13
Total	254		64		190		12		178		41		5		2		84		24		22	

CHART 26—NODULES (254)

| | Patients Seen | | | Evaluation Only | Entered Therapy | Inconclusive | Completed Therapy | Therapy | | | | | |
| | | | | | | | | Long-term | | | Short-term | | |
	M	F	Total					Excel.	Good	Fair	Excel.	Good	Fair
Totals	107	147	254	64	190	12	178	41	5	2	84	24	22
Percentage	42.1	57.9		25.2	74.8	6.3	93.7	23	2.8	1.1	47.2	13.5	12.4

| | Therapy Length Totals | | Therapy Results Totals | | |
	Long-term	Short-term	Excel.	Good	Fair
Totals	48	130	125	29	24
Percentage	27	73	70.2	16.3	13.5

CHART 27—POLYPS (68)

Age	Patients Seen M	F	Evaluation Only M	F	Entered Therapy M	F	Incon-clusive M	F	Completed Therapy M	F	Long-term Excel. M	F	Long-term Good M	F	Long-term Fair M	F	Short-term Excel. M	F	Short-term Good M	F	Short-term Fair M	F
0-10	1				1																1	1
11-20		3					1															1
21-30		8	1	3		2				2												
31-40	9	19	2	4	8	5	1		7	5	2	2					2	1	1	3	2	1
41-50	9	8	1	4	7	15		2	7	13	1	2		1			2	5	3	4		
51-60	6	4		1	5	4	1		4	4	1						3	4				
61-70		4				3				3											3	1
71+		1				1				1												
Subtotal	25	43	4	13	21	30	3	2	18	28	4	4		1			7	12	4	4	3	7
Total	68		17		51		5		46		8		1				19		8		10	

CHART 28—POLYPS (68)

	Patients Seen			Evaluation Only	Entered Therapy	Inconclusive	Completed Therapy	Therapy Long-term			Therapy Short-term		
	M	F	Total					Excel.	Good	Fair	Excel.	Good	Fair
Totals	25	43	68	17	51	5	46	8	1		19	8	10
Percentage	36.8	63.2		25	75	9.8	90.2	17.4	2.2		41.3	17.4	21.7

	Therapy Length Totals		Therapy Results Totals		
	Long-term	Short-term	Excel.	Good	Fair
Totals	9	37	27	9	10
Percentage	19.6	80.4	58.7	19.6	21.7

CHART 29—POLYPOID DEGENERATION (63)

Age	Patients Seen		Evaluation Only		Entered Therapy		Incon-clusive		Completed Therapy		Therapy											
											Long-term Excel.		Long-term Good		Long-term Fair		Short-term Excel.		Short-term Good		Short-term Fair	
	M	F	M	F	M	F	M	F	M	F	M	F	M	F	M	F	M	F	M	F	M	F
0-10																							
11-20	1				1				1								1					
21-30																							
31-40		7		4		3		1		2								2				
41-50	4	15		7	4	8		1	4	7	2						2	4		2		1
51-60	6	21	2	6	4	15		3	4	12		3		1			2	3		5	2	
61-70		6		4		2				2		1										1
71+	1	2			1	2			1	2		1					1	1				
Subtotal	12	51	2	21	10	30		5	10	25	2	5		1			6	10		7	2	2
Total	63		23		40		5		35		7		1				16		7		4	

CHART 30—POLYPOID DEGENERATION (63)

| | Patients Seen | | | Evaluation Only | Entered Therapy | Inconclusive Therapy | Completed Therapy | Therapy Long-term | | | Short-term | | |
	M	F	Total					Excel.	Good	Fair	Excel.	Good	Fair
Totals	12	51	63	23	40	5	35	7	1		16	7	4
Percentage	19	81		36.5	63.5	12.5	87.5	20	2.9		45.7	20	11.4

| | Therapy Length Totals | | Therapy Results Totals | | |
	Long-term	Short-term	Excel.	Good	Fair
Totals	8	27	23	8	4
Percentage	22.9	77.1	65.7	22.9	11.4

CHART 31—CONTACT ULCERS (85)

Note: The "Long-term" and "Short-term" result groups (Excel./Good/Fair) fall under the overall heading "Therapy."

Age	Patients Seen M	Patients Seen F	Evaluation Only M	Evaluation Only F	Entered Therapy M	Entered Therapy F	Incon-clusive M	Incon-clusive F	Completed Therapy M	Completed Therapy F	Long-term Excel. M	Long-term Excel. F	Long-term Good M	Long-term Good F	Long-term Fair M	Long-term Fair F	Short-term Excel. M	Short-term Excel. F	Short-term Good M	Short-term Good F	Short-term Fair M	Short-term Fair F
0-10																						
11-20	1	2		1	1	1		1	1		1											
21-30	8	3	3	1	8	2	2		6	2	2	1		1			3				1	
31-40	15	3	7	2	12	1			12	1	6	1					6					
41-50	24	8	4	1	17	7	2		15	7	7						4	6	3	1	1	
51-60	12	2	1	1	8	2			8	2	6						2	2				
61-70	1	1	3																			
71+	5				2				2								2					
Subtotal	66	19	18	6	48	13	4	1	44	12	22	2		1			17	8	3	1	2	
Total	85		24		61		5		56		24		1				25		4		2	

CHART 32—CONTACT ULCERS (85)

	Patients Seen			Evaluation Only	Entered Therapy	Inconclusive	Completed Therapy	Excel.	Therapy				
									Long-term		Short-term		
	M	F	Total						Good	Fair	Excel.	Good	Fair
Totals	66	19	85	24	61	5	56	24	1		25	4	2
Percentage	77.6	22.4		28.2	71.8	8.2	91.8	42.9	1.8		44.6	7.1	3.6

	Therapy Length Totals		Therapy Results Totals		
	Long-term	Short-term	Excel.	Good	Fair
Totals	25	31	49	5	2
Percentage	44.6	55.4	87.5	8.9	3.6

CHART 33—PAPILLOMATA (25)

Age	Patients Seen		Evaluation Only		Entered Therapy		Incon- clusive		Completed Therapy		Therapy											
											Long-term						Short-term					
											Excel.		Good		Fair		Excel.		Good		Fair	
	M	F	M	F	M	F	M	F	M	F	M	F	M	F	M	F	M	F	M	F	M	F
0-10	2	1		1	2		1		1				1									
11-20		3				3		1		2						2						
21-30		2				2		1		1												1
31-40	3	2		2	3		2		1												1	
41-50	6	2	3	1	3	1	1		2	1			1	1					1			
51-60																						
61-70	2	1	1		1	1			1	1						1					1	1
71+	1					1			1												1	
Subtotal	14	11	4	4	9	8	4	2	6	5			2	1		3			1		3	1
Total	25		8		17		6		11				3		3				1		4	

CHART 34—PAPILLOMATA (25)

	Patients Seen			Evaluation Only	Entered Therapy	Inconclusive Therapy	Completed Therapy	Therapy					
								Long-term			Short-term		
	M	F	Total					Excel.	Good	Fair	Excel.	Good	Fair
Totals	14	11	25	8	17	6	11		3	3		1	4
Percentage	56	44		32	68	35.3	64.7		27.3	27.3		9.1	36.4

	Therapy Length Totals		Therapy Results Totals		
	Long-term	Short-term	Excel.	Good	Fair
Totals	6	5		4	7
Percentage	54.5	45.5		36.4	63.6

CHART 35—LEUKOPLAKIA (17)

Age	Patients Seen M	F	Evaluation Only M	F	Entered Therapy M	F	Incon-clusive M	F	Completed Therapy M	F	Long-term Excel. M	F	Long-term Good M	F	Long-term Fair M	F	Short-term (Therapy) Excel. M	F	Short-term Good M	F	Short-term Fair M	F
0-10																						
11-20																						
21-30																						
31-40				1																		
41-50	4	1	3	1	1				1													
51-60	7	1	1	1	6		1		5		1				2							
61-70	3	1	1		2				2								1	2			1	1
71+																						
Subtotal	14	3	5	3	9		1		8		1				2		3				2	
Total	17		8		9		1		8		1				2		3				2	

CHART 36—LEUKOPLAKIA (17)

	Patients Seen			Evaluation Only	Entered Therapy	Inconclusive	Completed Therapy	Therapy					
	M	F	Total					Long-term			Short-term		
								Excel.	Good	Fair	Excel.	Good	Fair
Totals	14	3	17	8	9	1	8	1		2	3		2
Percentage	82.4	17.6		47.1	52.9	11.1	88.9	12.5		25	37.5		25

	Therapy Length Totals		Therapy Results Totals		
	Long-term	Short-term	Excel.	Good	Fair
Totals	3	5	4	4	4
Percentage	37.5	62.5	50	50	50

CHART 37—KERATOSIS (6)

Age	Patients Seen M	Patients Seen F	Evaluation Only M	Evaluation Only F	Entered Therapy M	Entered Therapy F	Incon-clusive M	Incon-clusive F	Completed Therapy M	Completed Therapy F	Long-term Excel. M	Long-term Excel. F	Long-term Good M	Long-term Good F	Long-term Fair M	Long-term Fair F	Short-term Excel. M	Short-term Excel. F	Short-term Good M	Short-term Good F	Short-term Fair M	Short-term Fair F
0-10																						
11-20																						
21-30		1				1				1										1		
31-40	1				1				1								1					
41-50	1				1				1		1											
51-60	1		1																			
61-70	1	1			1	1	1			1						1						
71+																						
Subtotal	4	2	1		3	2	1		2	2	1					1	1			1		
Total	6		1		5		1		4		1				1		1		1			

CHART 38—KERATOSIS(6)

| | Patients Seen | | | Evaluation Only | Entered Therapy | Inconclusive | Completed Therapy | Therapy | | | | | |
| | | | | | | | | Long-term | | | Short-term | | |
	M	F	Total				Excel.	Excel.	Good	Fair	Excel.	Good	Fair
Totals	4	2	6	1	5	1	4	1	1		1	1	1
Percentage	66.7	33.3		16.7	83.3	20	80	25	25		25	25	25

Therapy Length Totals

	Long-term	Short-term
Totals	2	2
Percentage	50	50

Therapy Results Totals

	Excel.	Good	Fair
Totals	2	1	1
Percentage	50	25	25

CHART 39—PARALYTIC DYSPHONIA (59)

Age	Patients Seen M	F	Evaluation Only M	F	Entered Therapy M	F	Incon-clusive M	F	Completed Therapy M	F	Long-term Excel. M	F	Long-term Good M	F	Long-term Fair M	F	Short-term Excel. M	F	Short-term Good M	F	Short-term Fair M	F
0-10																						
11-20	1	1	1			1				1				1								
21-30	2	3		2	2	1	2			1												1
31-40	6	3	3	1	3	2		1	3	1				1			1		1		1	
41-50	8	8	4	5	4	3			4	3	1						1	3	1		1	
51-60	8	11	4	5	4	6			4	6	2	3					1	1	1	1		1
61-70	2	5	1	4	1	1			1	1		1					1					
71+		1				1				1												1
Subtotal	27	32	13	17	14	15	2	1	12	14	3	4		2			4	4	3	1	2	3
Total	59		30		29		3		26		7		2				8		4		5	

CHART 40—PARALYTIC DYSPHONIA (59)

	Patients Seen			Evaluation Only	Entered Therapy	Inconclusive	Completed Therapy	Therapy					
								Long-term			Short-term		
	M	F	Total					Excel.	Good	Fair	Excel.	Good	Fair
Totals	27	32	59	30	29	3	26	7	2		8	4	5
Percentage	45.8	54.2		50.8	49.2	10.3	89.7	26.9	7.7		30.8	15.4	19.2

	Therapy Length Totals		Therapy Results Totals		
	Long-term	Short-term	Excel.	Good	Fair
Totals	9	17	15	6	5
Percentage	34.6	65.4	57.7	23.1	19.2

CHART 41—PARKINSON'S DISEASE (14)

Age	Patients Seen		Evaluation Only		Entered Therapy		Incon- clusive		Completed Therapy		Therapy											
											Long-term						Short-term					
											Excel.		Good		Fair		Excel.		Good		Fair		
	M	F	M	F	M	F	M	F	M	F	M	F	M	F	M	F	M	F	M	F	M	F
0-10																							
11-20																							
21-30																							
31-40																							
41-50	3	1	2		1	1	1			1				1									
51-60	2		1		1		1																
61-70	4		2		2				2													2	
71+	3	1	1	1	2		1		1							1							
Subtotal	12	2	6	1	6	1	3		3	1				1		1						2	
Total	14		7		7		3		4					1		1						2	

CHART 42—PARKINSON'S DISEASE (14)

| | Patients Seen | | | Evaluation Only | Entered Therapy | Inconclusive | Completed Therapy | Therapy | | | | | |
| | | | | | | | | Long-term | | | Short-term | | |
	M	F	Total					Excel.	Good	Fair	Excel.	Good	Fair
Totals	12	2	14	7	7	3	4		1	1			2
Percentage	85.7	14.3		50	50	42.9	57.1		25	25			50

| Therapy Length Totals | | | Therapy Results Totals | | |
Long-term	Short-term		Excel.	Good	Fair
2	2	Totals	1	1	3
50	50	Percentage	25	25	75

CHART 43—NEUROLOGICAL (33)

Age	Patients Seen M	Patients Seen F	Evaluation Only M	Evaluation Only F	Entered Therapy M	Entered Therapy F	Inconclusive M	Inconclusive F	Completed Therapy M	Completed Therapy F	Long-term Excel. M	Long-term Excel. F	Long-term Good M	Long-term Good F	Long-term Fair M	Long-term Fair F	Short-term Excel. M	Short-term Excel. F	Short-term Good M	Short-term Good F	Short-term Fair M	Short-term Fair F
0-10	2	3	2	1		2		2														
11-20	2	2	2	1		1				1												1
21-30		2				2		1		1								1				
31-40	1		1																			
41-50	4	3	2	3	2				2				2									
51-60	6	2	6			2				2										1		1
61-70	2	1	1		1	1			1	1											1	1
71+	1	2	1	2																		
Subtotal	18	15	15	7	3	8		3	3	5			2					1		1	1	3
Total	33		22		11				8				2				1		1		4	

(2 Long-term Inconclusive)

CHART 44—NEUROLOGICAL (33)

	Patients Seen			Evaluation Only	Entered Therapy	Inconclusive Therapy	Completed Therapy	Therapy Long-term			Therapy Short-term		
	M	F	Total					Excel.	Good	Fair	Excel.	Good	Fair
Totals	18	15	33	22	11	3	8		2		1	1	4
Percentage	54.5	45.5		66.7	33.3	27.3	72.7		25		12.5	12.5	50

	Therapy Length Totals		Therapy Results Totals		
	Long-term	Short-term	Excel.	Good	Fair
Totals	2	6	1	3	4
Percentage	25	75	12.5	37.5	50

CHART 45—PARTIAL CORDECTOMY (3), COMPLETE CORDECTOMY (5), HEMILARYNGECTOMY (5)

Age	Patients Seen		Evaluation Only		Entered Therapy		Incon-clusive		Completed Therapy		Therapy										
											Long-term						Short-term					
											Excel.		Good		Fair		Excel.		Good		Fair	
	M	F	M	F	M	F	M	F	M	F	M	F	M	F	M	F	M	F	M	F	M	F
0-10																							
11-20																							
21-30		2		2																			
31-40	1	3		1	1	2			1	2			1							1		1
41-50		1				1		1															
51-60	2				2				2				2										
61-70	3	1			3	1	1		2	1											2	1
71+																							
Subtotal	6	7		3	6	4	1	1	5	3			3							1	2	2
Total	13		3		10		2		8				3							1	4	

CHART 46—PARTIAL CORDECTOMY (3), COMPLETE CORDECTOMY (5), HEMILARYNGECTOMY (5)

	Patients Seen			Evaluation Only	Entered Therapy	Inconclusive Therapy	Completed Therapy	Therapy Long-term			Short-term		
	M	F	Total					Excel.	Good	Fair	Excel.	Good	Fair
Totals	6	7	13	3	10	2	8		3			1	4
Percentage	46.2	53.8		23.1	76.9	20	80		37.5			12.5	50

	Therapy Length Totals		Therapy Results Totals		
	Long-term	Short-term	Excel.	Good	Fair
Totals	3	5		4	4
Percentage	37.5	62.5		50	50

CHART 47—LARYNGECTOMY (ESOPHAGEAL VOICE) (55)

Age	Patients Seen M	F	Evaluation Only M	F	Entered Therapy M	F	Incon-clusive M	F	Completed Therapy M	F	Therapy Long-term Excel. M	F	Long-term Good M	F	Long-term Fair M	F	Short-term Excel. M	F	Short-term Good M	F	Short-term Fair M	F
0-10																						
11-20																						
21-30																						
31-40	1				1				1								1					
41-50	9	1		1	9				9								5		3		1	
51-60	19	3	6	3	13		3		10		3						4		2		1	
61-70	14	3	3	1	11	2	4		7	2			1				1		2		3	2
71+	5		1		4		3		1								1					
Subtotal	48	7	10	5	38	2	10		28	2	3		1				12		7		5	2
Total	55		15		40		10		30		3		1				12		7		7	

CHART 48—LARYNGECTOMY (ESOPHAGEAL VOICE) (55)

	Patients Seen			Evaluation Only	Entered Therapy	Inconclusive	Completed Therapy	Therapy Long-term			Therapy Short-term		
	M	F	Total					Excel.	Good	Fair	Excel.	Good	Fair
Totals	48	7	55	15	40	10	30	3	1		12	7	7
Percentage	87.3	12.7		27.3	72.7	25	75	10	3.3		40	23.3	23.3

	Therapy Length Totals		Therapy Results Totals		
	Long-term	Short-term	Excel.	Good	Fair
Totals	4	26	15	8	7
Percentage	13.3	86.7	50	26.7	23.3

PART 5
VOCAL REHABILITATION: OBSERVATIONS AND RESULTS

DIFFERENTIAL DIAGNOSIS OF VOCAL FOLD GROWTHS

The problem of differential diagnosis for various vocal fold growths involves three aspects: (1) pathological reports may differ on the same tissue; (2) clinical reports may differ from pathological reports; and (3) the nomenclature may differ between two laryngologists examining the same lesion. Clinical refers to a visual examination by a laryngologist; pathological refers to a report of biopsied tissue by a pathologist.

Fitz-Hugh, Smith, and Chiong (1958), in studying 300 consecutive cases, found differences between the clinical and pathological diagnoses and between two pathological diagnoses. In reviewing other reports, these authors (p. 481-482) write:

> For instance, Stewart (1957) does not mention laryngeal nodules in his 104 cases of benign tumors of the larynx, but does have 61 cases of "Inflammatory Polypus." Epstein (1957) and his associates diagnosed 283 cases of laryngeal polyps in a group of 366 benign tumors, believing polyps, nodules, and polypoidal degenerations to be histologically identical nonneoplastic swellings of the membranous vocal cords. Salinger (1956), on the other hand, found that his pathologists diagnosed no polyps and only three vocal nodules in a series of 232 consecutive laryngeal biopsies. Undoubtedly, in our survey, Epstein and Stewart would have classified the majority of our nodular cases as polyps. There are many variants of nodules and polyps which may be placed in either class, depending upon the impression of the pathologist, and which are essentially different manifestations of one and the same condition.

In conclusion, Fitz-Hugh, Smith, and Chiong (p. 493) state: "From our own material and that available in the literature, there is obviously much confusion in the nomenclature and histological interpretation of benign specimens from the vocal cords." They (p. 495) continue: "Certainly, one admonition is recommended, namely, 'laryngologist, know your pathologist.'"

Stewart (1957, pp. 718-719) from his own investigation, reports: "I might mention after my own examination of the mi-

271

croscopic material from these growths that there is a considerable divergence of opinion in the reports issued by different Pathologists."

Cunning (1950) finds frequent confusion exists in the diagnosis between a polyp and a papilloma. Salinger (1956) found a group of 17 cases which were clinically diagnosed as papilloma, but pathology reports indicated that only eight were papilloma. New and Erich (1938, p. 843) state: "Papillomas, of course, are more frequently encountered than any other true benign neoplasm and form 27 per cent of our total group of tumors." Stewart (1957, p. 724) differs: "Hitherto papillomata have been considered to be the most prolific form of laryngeal benign tumour and they may well be, but not from my figures." Fitz-Hugh, Smith, and Chiong (1958, p. 482) report: "From our study, we must consider the laryngeal nodule as the commonest chronic benign lesion of the vocal cords for which tissue is removed for diagnostic and therapeutic measures."

New and Erich (1938, p. 842) have found:

> No classification of benign laryngeal tumors is altogether satisfactory. Clinically, it is an impossibility to distinguish many of these tumors, because they bear such close resemblance one to another. The histogenesis of some is so obscure that a pathologic classification cannot be prepared with complete accuracy.

Salinger (1956) reviews 232 consecutive biopsies covering a three year period, comparing the preoperative clinical diagnosis with the laboratory reports. He (p. 186) states: "I was amazed to note that only exceptionally did the two agree."

Since the diagnosis of vocal fold growths may be divergent, as indicated by the above authors, a voice therapist may be experiencing more success (or lack of success) with certain types of growths than is indicated because of possible confusion in diagnosis. The voice therapist has no role in differential diagnosis; however, he should be aware of the problems and difficulties involved in this area.

MEDICOLEGAL ASPECTS OF VOICE DISORDERS

This author has seen several patients for vocal rehabilitation following automobile accidents in which the voice was affected.

Some of these cases experienced an alteration in voice caused by physical laryngeal changes, such as vocal fold paralysis or paresis, bowed vocal folds, hematoma, or other vocal fold growth(s). Other patients underwent a change in pitch and quality created by psychological trauma following the accident. These patients experienced one or more dysphonias including falsetto voice, hysterical aphonia, hysterical dysphonia, incipient spastic dysphonia, and spastic dysphonia.

In a few patients, case histories revealed that vocal misuse and abuse were present prior to the accident. The accident merely heightened the attention to the laryngeal area, accentuating a deep concern for the voice and its vocal health. Previously unrecognized negative vocal symptoms were now noted by the individual who felt that the vocal difficulty had been caused by the accident.

Cornut and Rebattu (1969) indicate that those evaluating the aftereffects of laryngeal trauma must take into consideration the socioprofessional consequences, such as the individual's profession, in determining the settlement. Werner-Kukuk and von Leden (1969, p. 171) discuss the effect of accidents on the larynx.

> This case further supports the contention that minor structural and functional changes in the larynx may give rise to a significant modification in the vocal quality for months or years, even after complete resolution of the clinical findings. There is no need to stress the medicolegal import of these observations.

Many other individuals have experienced voice disorders due to occupational demands upon the speaking voice. Teachers have been forced to use the speaking voice in adverse situations, such as talking over noise on playgrounds and in classrooms near airports and freeways. None of these teachers who have experienced dysphonias have had any training in the use of the speaking voice. The impairment or loss of the voice in these individuals is directly related to their occupational requirements.

Unfortunately, insurance coverage for vocal rehabilitation has been more frequent when the patient has experienced an organic lesion on the vocal folds. Those who were diagnosed as having functional misphonia have often been unable to receive financial remuneration. Only when the functional misphonia has progressed to a point where the individual has been seriously affected or unable to continue teaching or where organic dysphonia has developed has the individual been covered financially. Training of the speaking voice prior to or during employment would have prevented the voice disorder in almost all cases.

OCCUPATIONS AND VOICE DISORDERS

A predominance of voice disorders has been noted in certain occupations, such as teachers, singers, lawyers, and theologians by many writers, including Brodnitz (1954) and this author (Cooper, 1968, 1969b, 1970c-1970f, 1970h, 1970i, and 1970k). To determine the relationship between occupations and voice disorders, group of patients were reviewed to determine their occupations. These groups included all patients seen with functional misphonia (486), nodules (254), polyps (68), polypoid degeneration (63), and contact ulcers (85) for a total of 956 patients. The top 22 occupations are as follows:

1. Housewives (157)
2. Teachers (104)
3. Students (92)
4. Salespeople (68)
5. Owner/Manager (47)
6. Executives (46)
7. Singers (45)
8. Clerks (39)
9. Lawyers (32)
10. Engineers (32)
11. Actors/Actresses (24)
12. Theologians (24)
13. Secretaries (24)
14. Accountants (21)
15. Doctors (17)
16. Researchers (16)
17. Writers (15)
18. Public Relations (12)
19. Newscasters/announcers (11)
20. Telephone operators (11)
21. Music Teachers (10)
22. Social Workers (9)

Since vocal misuse causes functional misphonia, nodules, polyps, polypoid degeneration, and contact ulcers, a large number of persons from "talking" occupations would be anticipated. For the most part, these occupational groupings are mainly those in which the voice is used and apparently misused. In addition, a questionnaire was devised to elicit information regarding the use and misuse of the speaking voice from representative groups. (See Appendix C.) Three sets of results are included: from teachers—179 individuals, from theologians—267 individuals, and from the general public—432 individuals. (See Appendices

D, E, and F.) The teacher questionnaires were obtained in 1970 from a group of classroom teachers enrolled in a survey course on voice and speech disorders taught by the author. The theologian surveys were obtained in 1971 from two different meetings of theologians of 161 and 106 members respectively. The general public questionnaire involved three separate groups who were enrolled in voice improvement classes taught by the author in two successive years, 1970 (214 students and 60 students) and 1971 (158 students). An analysis of the results indicates the prevalence of voice problems in all of these groups as evidenced by the negative vocal symptoms.

RESULTS OF VOCAL REHABILITATION

In the literature, different voice therapists have indicated their criteria for evaluating the results of vocal rehabilitation. Brodnitz has one of the most complete discussions on this aspect. He (1963, p. 152) establishes the criteria in various categories to determine the results of vocal rehabilitation.

> As *successful*, those cases were listed where the patient, at the end of the treatment (whether vocal training alone or surgery followed by vocal rehabilitation) was able to produce a physiologically and esthetically satisfying voice what stands up well under all conditions of social and professional activities.
>
> As *improved*, those patients who emerge from the treatment with better and usable voices that still retain traces of the dysphonia.
>
> As *poor* results, those patients who in spite of a good surgical result and persistent therapeutic efforts are still left with a faulty voice.
>
> To those 3 groups a fourth one has to be added: The patients who do not accept the need for vocal rehabilitation or who discontinue treatment at an early stage.*

To evaluate the patients, Brodnitz (p. 151) says: "The trained ear of the phoniatrist is still the best means of determining the results of vocal rehabilitation." Flower (1959, p. 944) indicates his criteria: "Voice training was considered successful when a more acceptable voice was achieved and maintained, and when

---

* *Archives of Otolaryngology,* 77:152, 1963. Copyright 1963, American Medical Association.

there was no evidence of misuse on laryngeal examination at the six months' recheck."

To more fully understand and to discuss the voice patients seen, this author devised a system in which each patient seen was categorized and/or evaluated. The following chart indicates the subdivisions as described below:

Patients Seen

Evaluation Only   Entered Therapy

Inconclusive   Completed Therapy

Long-term   Short-term

Excellent Good Fair   Excellent Good Fair

All patients were counted under the heading Patients Seen. This major category of the total number of patients seen was subgrouped into two divisions: the number seen for Evaluation Only (one to two sessions) and the number who Entered Therapy. In the second division, those entering therapy were further broken down into two additional groupings: the number judged Inconclusive (discontinuing therapy after a minimal number of sessions) and the number who Completed Therapy. Those who were termed inconclusive were judged as such by the voice therapist; these patients, although they may have been making excellent or good progress, did not complete therapy. Most patients who were inconclusive had received short-term therapy, usually discontinuing therapy after a limited number of sessions. A few patients, approximately nine out of the total group, were considered inconclusive after having received long-term therapy, since at the termination of their therapy they had made less than fair improvement. These patients were in the categories of spastic dysphonia (4 patients), ventricular phonation (3 patients), and other neurological disorders (2 patients), which represent the voice disorders that are the most difficult to overcome. Therapy in most of these cases was terminated by the therapist who decided that the patient, for one reason or another, was not progressing and would not progress.

The two therapy lengths which have been designated were short-term therapy and long-term therapy. Short-term therapy refers to therapy which lasted six months or less. Long-term therapy refers to therapy which lasted over six months.

For those patients completing vocal rehabilitation, general criteria were established to judge the results of vocal therapy as being excellent, good, or fair. These general criteria were based on the three groupings of the negative vocal symptoms: sensory, auditory, and visual. The patient alone determined the sensory judgement; the patient and the therapist together evaluated the auditory aspect; the laryngologist made the visual evaluation. Since some patients may have experienced impairment in only one or two of the three symptom groupings, the general criteria are relative and were individually applied to each patient. The ultimate judgement of the therapy results was based on each patient's original vocal impairment as compared to the final outcome of vocal rehabilitation in one or more of these modalities. Some patients who are listed as completing therapy with fair results and still other patients who were considered inconclusive could have possibly experienced good or excellent results had they remained in therapy longer.

GENERAL CRITERIA FOR PATIENTS COMPLETING VOCAL REHABILITATION

Symptoms	Excellent	Good	Fair
Sensory	Absence of laryngeal or pharyngeal pain, discomfort, or irritation during and after speaking.	Slight pain, irritation, or discomfort during or after speaking.	Some pain, irritation or discomfort during or after speaking.
Auditory	Automaticity of correct pitch, tone focus, quality, volume, breath support, and rate in spontaneous speech 90-100% of the time.	Automaticity of vocal variables in spontaneous speech 80-90% of the time.	Automaticity of vocal variables in spontaneous speech 70-80% of the time.
Visual	Absence of inflammation and/or lesion(s); cords normal in appearance with smooth approximation during phonation.	Slight inflammation occasionally; cords essentially normal in appearance with smooth approximation during most phonation.	Some inflammation; reduction of lesion; improvement in the approximation of cords during phonation.

The above criteria do not completely apply for patients experiencing paralytic dysphonia, Parkinson's disease, other neurological disorders, partial cordectomy, complete cordectomy, hemilaryngectomy, and laryngectomy. The auditory symptoms are the most relevant; the sensory symptoms are of less relevance; and the visual symptoms as described in the chart are not essentially applicable.

For a more revealing discussion and a more comprehensive understanding of the results, patients with functional misphonia and the organic dysphonias of nodules, polyps, polypoid degeneration, and contact ulcers were further grouped into various categories. The purpose of these groupings was to determine which categories of patients were most likely to enter therapy and were most likely to complete therapy.

All of these patients were divided into private patients and clinic patients. Private patients were those individuals seen as private patients by the referring physicians. Clinic patients were those individuals seen in the UCLA medical clinic by physicians on the medical staff and by residents.

A further classification of patients with functional misphonia was the length of time which the patient had had the dysphonia. This has been indicated by short-term onset and long-term onset. Short-term onset was six months or less; long-term onset was over six months. This classification was not applied to patients with the organic dysphonias, since the onset was considered to be long-term in almost all cases.

Patients who had the organic vocal fold lesions of nodules, polyps, polypoid degeneration, and contact ulcers were divided into three groupings. The three groups were (1) "postoperative" patients who had surgery (one or more times) to remove the lesion(s) prior to vocal rehabilitation; the lesion was not present when therapy began; (2) "postoperative and return" patients who had surgery (one or more times) for removal of the lesion which was followed by a return of the lesion(s) (one or more times); the lesion(s) was present when therapy began; and (3) "no surgery" patients who had not had surgery prior to vocal rehabilitation; the lesion(s) was present when therapy began.

The totals and percentages of each dysphonia seen are shown in Chart A. The most frequently seen dysphonias were functional misphonia, 486 patients or 34.6 percent; nodules, 254 patients or 18.1 percent; contact ulcers, 85 patients or 6 percent; polyps, 68 patients or 4.8 percent; polypoid degeneration, 63 patients or 4.5 percent; spastic dysphonia and incipient spastic dysphonia, 63 patients or 4.5 percent; and paralytic dysphonia, 59 patients or 4.2 percent. The other dysphonias seen were under 4 percent of the total seen.

Of the 1406 total patients seen in all categories, 954 or 67.9 percent entered therapy and 836 or 87.6 percent completed therapy. Of the 693 patients seen with functional dysphonias, 467 or 67.4 percent entered therapy and 408 or 87.4 percent completed therapy. Of the 658 patients seen with organic dysphonias (omitting laryngectomy), 447 or 67.9 percent entered therapy and 398 or 89 percent completed therapy. Comparing the therapy lengths of functional and organic dysphonias, 84 patients or 20.6 percent of functional dysphonic patients and 125 patients or 31.4 percent of organic dysphonic patients had long-term therapy. Short-term therapy for functional dysphonias involved 324 patients or 79.4 percent and for organic dysphonias involved 273 patients or 68.6 percent. In comparing the therapy results, excellent was designated for 299 or 73.3 percent of functional dysphonias and for 254 or 63.8 percent of organic dysphonias. Good was judged for 73 or 17.9 percent of functional dysphonias and for 75 or 18.8 percent of organic dysphonias. Fair was designated for 36 or 8.8 percent of functional dysphonias and for 69 or 17.3 percent of organic dysphonias. (See Chart B for complete results.)

Patients experiencing functional misphonia and organic dysphonia (nodules, polyps, polypoid degeneration and contact ulcers) are fully described in Charts C and D. Conclusions which may be noted from these break-downs are as follows:

1. Of 486 functional misphonic patients seen and 470 organic dysphonic patients seen, 341 or 70.2 percent of functional misphonic patients and 342 or 72.8 percent of organic dysphonic patients entered therapy. Of these groups, 313 or 91.8 percent of functional misphonic patients and 315 or 92.1 percent of organic dysphonic patients completed therapy.

2. In comparing private and clinic patients, in those patients with functional misphonia, of the 408 private patients and 78

clinic patients seen, 291 or 71.3 percent of the private patients and 50 or 64.1 percent of the clinic patients entered therapy. Of these groups entering therapy, 275 or 94.5 percent of the private patients and 38 or 78 percent of the clinic patients completed therapy. In those patients with organic dysphonia, of the 390 private patients and 80 clinic patients seen, 289 or 74.1 percent of the private patients and 53 or 66.3 percent of the clinic patients entered therapy. Of these groups entering therapy, 274 or 94.8 percent of the private patients and 41 or 77.4 percent of the clinic patients completed therapy.

3. In comparing the length of onset for functional misphonic patients, of the 457 long-term onset patients and 29 short-term onset patients seen, 322 or 70.5 percent of the long-term onset patients and 19 or 65.5 percent of the short-term onset patients entered therapy. Of these groups entering therapy, 295 or 91.6 percent of the long-term onset patients and 18 or 94.7 percent of the short-term onset patients completed therapy.

4. In comparing the groups within organic dysphonia, of the 180 postoperative patients seen, 135 or 75 percent entered therapy and 123 or 91.1 percent completed therapy; of the 66 postoperative and return patients seen, 49 or 74.2 percent entered therapy and 44 or 89.8 percent completed therapy; of the 224 no surgery patients seen, 158 or 70.5 percent entered therapy and 148 or 93.7 percent completed therapy.

An abbreviated summation is as follows:

1. Of the total functional misphonic patients seen, 70.2 percent entered therapy and 91.8 percent completed therapy. Of the total organic dysphonic patients seen, 72.8 percent entered therapy and 92.1 percent completed therapy.

2. Of the total private patients seen with functional misphonia, 71.3 percent entered therapy and 94.5 percent completed therapy. Of the total private patients seen with organic dysphonia, 74.1 percent entered therapy and 94.8 percent completed therapy.

3. Of the total clinic patients seen with functional misphonia, 64.1 percent entered therapy and 78 percent completed therapy. Of the total clinic patients seen with organic dysphonia, 66.3 percent entered therapy and 77.4 percent completed therapy.

4. Of the long-term onset patients seen (functional misphonia), 70.5 percent entered therapy and 91.6 percent completed therapy. Of the short-term onset patients seen (functional misphonia), 65.5 percent entered therapy and 94.7 percent completed therapy.

5. Of the total postoperative patients seen (organic dysphonia), 75 percent entered therapy and 91.1 percent completed therapy. Of the total postoperative and return patients seen (organic dysphonia), 74.2 percent entered therapy and 89.8 percent completed therapy. Of the total no surgery patients seen (organic dysphonia), 70.5 percent entered therapy and 93.7 percent completed therapy.

Concerning the results of therapy and the length of therapy in relation to other factors, the following conclusions may be observed:

1. The majority of patients completing therapy achieved excellent results: functional misphonia, 74.4 percent and organic dysphonia, 71.1 percent.

2. The majority of patients were seen for short-term therapy: functional misphonia, 83.7 percent and organic dysphonia, 71.4 percent.

3. Out of the 341 functional misphonic patients entering therapy and the 342 organic dysphonic patients entering therapy, only 8.2 percent of functional misphonic and 7.9 percent of the organic dysphonic were inconclusive.

4. All functional misphonic patients with short-term onset required only short-term therapy, except one patient.

5. Long-term therapy has a very high percentage of excellent results. In functional misphonia, 45 out of 51 long-term therapy patients (88.2%) were excellent; in organic dysphonia, 80 out of 90 long-term therapy patients (88.9%) were excellent.

6. Private patients were seen more often for long-term therapy (functional misphonia, 16.7%; organic dysphonia, 30.3%) than were clinic patients (functional misphonia, 13.3%; organic dysphonia, 82.9%).

7. Clinic patients were seen more often for short-term therapy (functional misphonia, 86.8%; organic dysphonia, 82.9%) than were private patients (functional misphonia, 83.3%; organic dysphonia, 69.7%).

8. Private patients were more likely to achieve excellent results (functional misphonia, 77.1% and organic dysphonia, 73.4%) than were clinic patients (functional misphonia, 55.3% and organic dysphonia, 56.1%).

9. Clinic patients were more likely to be judged good or fair (*good:* functional misphonia, 34.2%; organic dysphonia, 24.4% and *fair:* functional misphonia, 10.5%; organic dysphonia, 19.5%) than were private patients (*good:* functional misphonia, 14.5%; organic dysphonia, 15% and *fair:* functional misphonia, 8.4%; organic dysphonia, 11.7%).

10. Postoperative patients and no surgery patients (no lesion present in these two groups) were seen for short-term therapy (postoperative, 76.4% and no surgery, 72.3%) more often than postoperative and return patients, 54.5 percent (lesion present).

11. Of the postoperative patients, 74.4 percent had had only one surgery and 25.6 percent had had two or more. Of the postoperative patients, only 47 percent had had one surgery while 53 percent had had two or more surgeries.

12. Postoperative and return patients were more likely to achieve excellent results (79.5%), followed by no surgery patients (73.6%), than were postoperative patients (65%).

13. Of the 246 patients seen who had had surgery (postoperative, 180; postoperative and return, 66), 165 or 67.1 percent had had one surgery and 81 or 32.9 percent had had two or more surgeries.

For a more detailed review of the individual organic lesions, Charts E, F, G and H may be examined. These four charts were combined to make Chart D.

FOLLOW-UP RESULTS OF VOCAL REHABILITATION

A follow-up of patients who have completed therapy is an important and vital aspect of vocal rehabilitation. There are few clinical follow-up studies of voice cases in the literature. Among these are Flower (1959), Peacher (1961), and Brodnitz (1963).

Flower (1959) uses a six months' follow-up laryngeal examination to determine if misuse is present and considers the achievement and maintenance of an acceptable voice to be an indication of successful voice training. Peacher (1961) was able to follow 70 contact ulcer patients (out of 101 patients seen for vocal therapy) from one to twelve years following therapy. Peacher uses as criteria the recurrence or nonrecurrence of the contact ulcer; 65 out of the 70 patients had not experienced a recurrence. Brodnitz (1963, p. 155) finds that 145 patients or 40 percent of the successfully treated patients with functional voice disorders (which includes nodules, polyps, polypoid thickening, and contact ulcers) "were found to be in good voices and free of recurrences." These patients were observed over varying periods of one to eight years.

In this follow-up study, letters were sent to patients who had completed therapy with excellent, good, and fair results. The letters requested (1) a self-rating of the patient's voice at the present time based on symptomatology and laryngeal examination; (2) the length of time since therapy had been concluded; and (3) a request for the patient to contact the therapist for a follow-up evaluation of the voice (without charge to the patient).

This therapist was personally able to evaluate 101 patients; an additional 144 patients replied to the letter only. To determine the validity of the self-rating of these 144 patients whom the therapist was unable to rate, a comparison has been made between the therapist's and patient's ratings in the 101 patients. This comparison, which is shown in Chart I, shows agreement between the therapist and the patient in 93 ratings or 92.1 percent. The patient's self-rating is higher in 5 or 5 percent and lower in 3 or 3 percent than the therapist's rating. In view of this high percentage of agreement between therapist and patient ratings, the self-ratings of the other 144 patients would appear to be valid. Thus, a total of 245 patients are included in the follow-up.

The length of time between completion of therapy and the follow-up ranged from six months to ten years, as shown in Chart J. The average length of time was approximately two years and seven months.

Of the 245 patients in the follow-up, 129 had experienced functional dysphonias and 116 had had organic dysphonias. An

analysis of the individual types of functional and organic dysphonias is shown in Chart K.

To determine the lasting success of vocal rehabilitation, the
results obtained at the end of therapy were compared to the follow-up results, as shown in Chart L. Of the 245 patients, 233 patients or 95.1 percent had a follow-up rating of excellent or
good; these patients were considered to have retained their vocal
recovery or, in a few cases, to have continued to improve following the completion of therapy. The other 12 patients or 4.9
percent remained fair or regressed. It should be noted that 73
patients or 29.8 percent moved from excellent to good; however,
a rating of good is indicative of the retention of vocal recovery.
This slight regression also indicates that periodic therapy check-
ups following the completion of therapy appears essential to
prevent any regression. This follow-up indicates the stability of
successful vocal rehabilitation.

PREVENTIVE VOCAL REHABILITATION

Preventive medicine is an accepted fact today, but where is
preventive voice therapy? We have, essentially, no professor of
preventive vocal rehabilitation; we are not concerned with the
prevention of voice problems. We are concerned essentially with
existing severe functional and organic dysphonias.

Elementary and high schools have no meaningful programs
of vocal hygiene or training the speaking voice which would be
designed to prevent voice problems. Universities and colleges are
without programs that would develop and train the speaking
voice for those professionals, such as teachers, lawyers, and physicians, who need and use the speaking voice routinely. Classes
in public speaking are not classes in voice training.

Another aspect of the problem lies within the educational
training of laryngologists. Laryngologists may not be given
training in recognizing a misused voice that has no organic lesion on the vocal folds nor in understanding the fact that vocal
misuse may lead to functional misphonia and eventually to organic dysphonias. Tarneaud (1958), Moses (1948), and Ferguson (1955), among other laryngologists, have indicated aspects
of this situation. Ferguson (1955, p. 327) writes:

Laryngologists have long admitted that organic lesions of the larynx may be produced by mis-use of the voice, but few among us really know what actually constitutes mis-use of the voice, or how to correct it. Diagnosis and management of patients afflicted with these lesions would benefit enormously from a sound knowledge of the methods and principles of voice production. Even though none of us expect to qualify as teachers of voice, we should train our ears to perceive vocal strain and to recognize the physical and mental symptoms which attend this difficulty.

Preventive vocal rehabilitation has been discussed and recommended for many years. Froeschels (1943) suggests using the chewing method in kindergartens, grammar schools, high schools, universities, and professional groups to avoid voice problems. Kallen (1959) discusses the need to train the voice from childhood through puberty until the adult voice is established. He advises preventive care for those individuals who need to use their voices professionally. Brodnitz (1962) also notes the need for training the voice for professional people. Peacher (1952, p. 14) states:

> Second, there is another thing that we may do in the way of prevention. Vocal training in schools leading to professions where speaking is very important. It is needed in the schools of theology, law, business, government, medicine, teaching, etc.

Glasgow (1944) writes that teachers should have voice training. Anderson (1944) notes that 29 percent of a group of 1200 prospective teachers had voice problems. Preventive voice training programs for teachers have been discussed by Labastida (1961), Lejska (1967), Gundermann (1963), Gundermann, Weuffen, and Luth (1966), and Pahn and Glatz (1969).

Since many physicians and the general population are uninformed about voice disorders, the voice therapist should make these individuals aware of dysphonias as a public service and public education. Vocal misuse and vocal suicide would be less frequent if people were informed about voice disorders and vocal rehabilitation.

Until the medical profession makes its members and students aware of vocal rehabilitation, until the school systems train students meaningfully and pertinently in using the speaking voice, and until the colleges and universities establish a program of vocal training for professionals who use their voices routinely, many individuals will incur voice disorders that are accepted as normal. We must always be concerned with vocal rehabilitation, but we also need to always be concerned with the prevention of dysphonias.

CHART A

TOTALS AND PERCENTAGES OF EACH DYSPHONIA SEEN

		%
Functional misphonia	486	34.6
Falsetto	34	2.4
Ventricular phonation	11	.8
Hysterical aphonia	9	.6
Hysterical dysphonia	9	.6
Functional aphonia	5	.4
Spastic dysphonia	42	3.0
Incipient spastic dysphonia	21	1.5
Nasality—functional	44	3.1
Nasality—organic	11	.8
Bowed vocal folds—functional	32	2.3
Bowed vocal folds—organic	10	.7
Nodules	254	18.1
Polyps	68	4.8
Polypoid degeneration	63	4.5
Contact ulcers	85	6.1
Papillomata	25	1.8
Leukoplakia	17	1.2
Keratosis	6	.4
Paralytic dysphonia	59	4.2
Parkinson's disease	14	1.0
Other neurological	33	2.3
Partial cordectomy, complete cordectomy, hemilaryngectomy	13	.9
Laryngectomy	55	3.9
Total	1406	

CHART B—TOTAL PATIENTS SEEN

	Patients Seen				Total	Evaluation Only	%	Entered Therapy	%	Incon-clusive	%	Completed Therapy	%
	Male	%	Female	%									
Functional misphonia	244	50.2	242	49.8	486	145	29.8	341	70.2	28	8.2	313	91.8
Falsetto	30	88.2	4	11.8	34	12	35.3	22	64.7	2	9.1	20	90.9
Ventricular phonation	4	36.4	7	63.6	11	5	45.5	6	54.5	3	50	3	50
Hysterical aphonia	1	11.1	8	88.9	9	4	44.4	5	55.6	1	20	4	80
Hysterical dysphonia	2	22.2	7	77.8	9	3	33.3	6	66.7			6	100
Functional aphonia	1	20	4	80	5			5	100			5	100
Spastic dysphonia	18	42.9	24	57.1	42	20	47.6	22	52.4	16	72.7	6	27.3
Incipient spastic dysphonia	7	33.3	14	66.7	21	8	38.1	13	61.9	4	30.8	9	69.2
Nasality—functional	23	52.3	21	47.7	44	23	52.3	21	47.7	3	14.3	18	85.7
Nasality—organic	5	45.5	6	54.5	11	4	36.4	7	63.6			7	100
Bowed vocal folds functional	20	62.5	12	37.5	32	6	18.75	26	81.25	2	7.7	24	92.3
organic	3	30	7	70	10			10	100	3	30	7	70
Nodules	107	42.1	147	57.9	254	64	25.2	190	74.8	12	6.3	178	93.7
Polyps	25	36.8	43	63.2	68	17	25	51	75	5	9.8	46	90.2
Polypoid degeneration	12	19	51	81	63	23	36.5	40	63.5	5	12.5	35	87.5
Contact ulcers	66	77.6	19	22.4	85	24	28.2	61	71.8	5	8.2	56	91.8
Papillomata	14	56	11	44	25	8	32	17	68	6	35.3	11	64.7
Leukoplakia	14	82.4	3	17.6	17	8	47.1	9	52.9	1	11.1	8	88.9
Keratosis	4	66.7	2	33.3	6	1	16.7	5	83.3	1	20	4	80
Paralytic dysphonia	27	45.8	32	54.2	59	30	50.8	29	49.2	3	10.3	26	89.7
Parkinson's disease	12	85.7	2	14.3	14	7	50	7	50	3	42.9	4	57.1
Other neurological	18	54.5	15	45.5	33	22	66.7	11	33.3	3	27.3	8	72.7
Partial cordectomy, complete cordectomy, hemilaryngectomy	6	46.2	7	53.8	13	3	23.1	10	76.9	2	20	8	80
Laryngectomy	48	87.3	7	12.7	55	15	27.3	40	72.7	10	25	30	75
Total	711	50.6	695	49.4	1406	452	32.1	954	67.9	118	12.4	836	87.6
Functional total	350	50.5	343	49.5	693	226	32.6	467	67.4	59	12.6	408	87.4
Organic total (omitting laryngectomy)	313	47.6	345	52.4	658	211	32.1	447	67.9	49	11	398	89.0

CHART B (Continued)—TOTAL PATIENTS SEEN

	Long-Term Therapy						Short-Term Therapy					
	Excel.	%	Good	%	Fair	%	Excel.	%	Good	%	Fair	%
Functional misphonia	45	14.4	5	1.6	1	.3	188	60.1	48	15.3	26	8.3
Falsetto	3	15	1	5	1	5	12	60	1	5	2	10
Ventricular phonation	1	33.3					1	33.3	1	33.3		
Hysterical aphonia							3	75	1	25		
Hysterical dysphonia	1	16.7					3	50	2	33.3		
Functional aphonia							5	100				
Spastic dysphonia	1	16.7	3	50	2	33.3						
Incipient spastic dysphonia	2	22.2			1	11.1	4	44.4	2	22.2		
Nasality—functional	7	38.9	2	11.1	1	5.6	3	16.7	5	27.8		
Nasality—organic	2	28.6	2	28.6	1	14.3	1	14.3	1	14.3		
Bowed vocal folds functional	7	29.2					13	54.2	2	8.3	2	8.3
organic	2	28.6	1	14.3			3	42.9				
Nodules	41	23	5	2.8	2	1.1	84	47.2	24	13.5	22	12.4
Polyps	8	17.4	1	2.2			19	41.3	8	17.4	10	21.7
Polypoid degeneration	7	20	1	2.9			16	45.7	7	20	4	11.4
Contact ulcers	24	42.9	1	1.8			25	44.6	4	7.1	2	3.6
Papillomata			3	27.3	3	27.3			1	9.1	4	36.4
Leukoplakia	1	12.5			2	25	3	37.5	2	25		
Keratosis	1	25			1	25	1	25			1	25
Paralytic dysphonia	7	26.9	2	7.7			8	30.8	4	15.4	5	19.2
Parkinson's disease			1	25	1	25					2	50
Other neurological			2	25			1	12.5	1	12.5	4	50
Partial cordectomy, complete cordectomy, hemilaryngectomy			3	37.5			1	12.5	1	12.5		
Laryngectomy	3	10	1	3.3			12	40	7	23.3	7	23.3
Total	163	19.5	34	4.1	16	1.9	405	48.4	122	14.6	96	11.5
Functional—total	67	16.4	11	2.7	6	1.5	232	56.9	62	15.2	30	7.4
Organic total (omitting laryngectomy)	93	23.4	22	5.5	10	2.5	161	40.5	53	13.3	59	14.8

CHART B (Continued)—TOTAL PATIENTS SEEN

	Therapy Length Totals				Therapy Results Total					
	Long-Term	%	Short-Term	%	Excellent	%	Good	%	Fair	%
Functional misphonia	51	16.3	262	83.7	233	74.4	53	16.9	27	8.6
Falsetto	5	25	15	75	15	75	2	10	3	15
Ventricular phonation	1	33.3	2	66.7	2	66.7	1	33.3		
Hysterical aphonia			4	100	3	75	1	25		
Hysterical dysphonia	1	16.7	5	83.3	4	66.7	2	33.3		
Functional aphonia			5	100	5	100				
Spastic dysphonia	6	100			1	16.7	3	50	2	33.3
Incipient spastic dysphonia	3	33.3	6	66.7	6	66.7	2	22.2	1	11.1
Nasality—functional	10	55.6	8	44.4	10	55.6	7	38.9	1	5.6
Nasality—organic	5	71.4	2	28.6	3	42.8	3	42.8	1	14.3
Bowed vocal folds functional	7	29.2	17	70.8	20	83.3	2	8.3	2	8.3
organic	3	42.9	4	57.1	5	71.4	2	28.6		
Nodules	48	27	130	73	125	70.2	29	16.3	24	13.5
Polyps	9	19.6	37	80.4	27	58.7	9	19.6	10	21.7
Polypoid degeneration	8	22.9	27	77.1	23	65.7	8	22.9	4	11.4
Contact ulcers	25	44.6	31	55.4	49	87.5	5	8.9	2	3.6
Papillomata	6	54.5	5	45.5			4	36.4	7	63.6
Leukoplakia	3	37.5	5	62.5	4	50			4	50
Keratosis	2	50	2	50	2	50	1	25	1	25
Paralytic dysphonia	9	34.6	17	65.4	15	57.7	6	23.1	5	19.2
Parkinson's disease	2	50	2	50			1	25	3	75
Other neurological	2	25	6	75	1	12.5	3	37.5	4	50
Partial cordectomy, complete cordectomy, hemilaryngectomy	3	37.5	5	62.5			4	50		
Laryngectomy	4	13.3	26	86.7	15	50	8	26.7	7	23.3
Total	213	25.5	623	74.5	568	67.9	156	18.7	112	13.4
Functional—total	84	20.6	324	79.4	299	73.3	73	17.9	36	8.8
Organic total (omitting laryngectomy)	125	31.4	273	68.6	254	63.8	75	18.8	69	17.3

CHART C—FUNCTIONAL MISPHONIA

	Patients Seen	Evaluation Only	%	Entered Therapy	%	Inconclusive	%	Completed Therapy	%
Private	408	117	28.7	291	71.3	16	5.5	275	94.5
Clinic	78	28	35.9	50	64.1	12	24	38	78
Total	486	145	29.8	341	70.2	28	8.2	313	91.8
Length of onset (Private & Clinic)									
Long-term	457	135	29.5	322	70.5	27	8.4	295	91.6
Short-term	29	10	34.5	19	65.5	1	5.3	18	94.7

CHART C (Continued)—FUNCTIONAL MISPHONIA

	Long-term Therapy						Short-term Therapy					
	Excel.	%	Good	%	Fair	%	Excel.	%	Good	%	Fair	%
Private	40	14.5	5	1.8	1	.4	172	62.5	35	12.7	22	8.0
Clinic	5	13.2					16	42.1	13	34.2	4	10.5
Total	45	14.4	5	1.6	1	.3	188	60.1	48	15.3	26	8.3
Length of onset (Private & Clinic)												
Long-term	45	15.3	4	1.4	1	.3	174	58.9	47	15.9	24	8.1
Short-term			1	5.6			14	77.8	1	5.6	2	11.1

CHART C (*Continued*)—FUNCTIONAL MISPHONIA

| | Therapy Length Totals | | | | Therapy Results Totals | | | | | |
	Long-term	%	Short-term	%	Excel.	%	Good	%	Fair	%
Private	46	16.7	229	83.3	212	77.1	40	14.5	23	8.4
Clinic	5	13.2	33	86.8	21	55.3	13	34.2	4	10.5
Total	51	16.3	262	83.7	233	74.4	53	16.9	27	8.6
Length of onset (Private & Clinic)										
Long-term	50	16.9	245	83.1	219	74.2	51	17.3	25	8.5
Short-term	1	5.6	17	94.4	14	77.8	2	11.1	2	11.1

CHART D—ORGANIC DYSPHONIA (NODULES, POLYPS, POLYPOID DEGENERATION, CONTACT ULCERS)

	Patients Seen	Evaluation Only	%	Entered Therapy	%	Inconclusive	%	Completed Therapy	%
Private	390	101	25.9	289	74.1	15	5.2	274	94.8
Clinic	80	27	33.8	53	66.3	12	22.6	41	77.4
Private:									
Postoperative	150	36	24	114	78	7	6.1	107	93.9
PO* and return	57	15	26.3	42	73.7	3	7.1	39	92.9
No surgery	183	50	27.3	133	72.7	5	3.8	128	96.2
Clinic:									
Postoperative	30	9	30	21	70	5	23.8	16	76.2
PO* and return	9	2	22.2	7	77.8	2	28.6	5	71.4
No surgery	41	16	3.9	25	61	5	20	20	80
Private and clinic:									
Postoperative	180	45	25	135	75	12	8.9	123	91.1
PO* and return	66	17	25.8	49	74.2	5	10.2	44	89.8
No surgery	224	66	29.5	158	70.5	10	6.3	148	93.7
Total	470	128	27.2	342	72.8	27	7.9	315	92.1

* Postoperative

CHART D *(Continued)*—ORGANIC DYSPHONIA (NODULES, POLYPS, POLYPOID DEGENERATION, CONTACT ULCERS)

| | Long-term Therapy | | | | | | Short-term Therapy | | | | | |
	Excel.	%	Good	%	Fair	%	Excel.	%	Good	%	Fair	%
Private	73	26.6	8	2.9	2	.7	128	46.7	33	12.0	30	10.9
Clinic	7	17.1					16	39.0	10	24.4	8	19.5
Private:												
Postoperative	22	20.6	4	3.7	1	.9	50	46.7	16	15	14	13.1
PO* and return	17	43.6			1	2.6	14	35.9	3	7.7	4	10.3
No surgery	34	26.6	4	3			64	50	14	10.9	12	9.4
Clinic:												
Postoperative	2	12.5					6	37.5	2	12.5	6	37.5
PO* and return	2	40					2	40			1	20
No surgery	3	15					8	40	8	40	1	5
Private and clinic:												
Postoperative	24	19.5	4	3.3	1	.8	56	45.5	18	14.6	20	16.3
PO* and return	19	43.2			1	2.3	16	36.4	3	6.8	5	11.4
No surgery	37	25	4	2.7			72	48.6	22	14.9	13	8.8
Total	80	25.4	8	2.5	2	.6	144	45.7	43	13.7	38	12.1

* Postoperative

CHART D (Continued)—ORGANIC DYSPHONIA (NODULES, POLYPS, POLYPOID DEGENERATION, CONTACT ULCERS)

| | Therapy Length Totals | | | | Therapy Results Totals | | | | | |
	Long-term	%	Short-term	%	Excel.	%	Good	%	Fair	%
Private	83	30.3	191	69.7	201	73.4	41	15	32	11.7
Clinic	7	17.1	34	82.9	23	56.1	10	24.4	8	19.5
Private:										
Postoperative	27	25.2	80	74.8	72	67.3	20	18.7	15	14
PO* and return	18	46.2	21	53.8	31	79.5	3	7.7	5	12.8
No surgery	38	29.7	90	70.3	98	76.6	18	14.1	12	9.4
Clinic:										
Postoperative	2	12.5	14	87.5	8	50	2	12.5	6	37.5
PO* and return	2	40	3	60	4	80			1	20
No surgery	3	15	17	85	11	55	8	40	1	50
Private and clinic:										
Postoperative	29	23.6	94	76.4	80	65	22	17.9	21	17.1
PO* and return	20	45.5	24	54.5	35	79.5	3	6.8	6	13.6
No surgery	41	27.7	107	72.3	109	73.6	26	17.6	13	8.8
Total	90	28.6	225	71.4	224	71.1	51	16.2	40	12.7

* Postoperative

CHART D (*Continued*)—ORGANIC DYSPHONIA (NODULES, POLYPS, POLYPOID DEGENERATION, CONTACT ULCERS)

	Number of Surgeries				Total Patients Having Surgery		Total Patients Seen
	1	%	2+	%		%	
Private	137	66.2	70	33.8	207	53.1†	390
Clinic	28	71.8	11	28.2	39	48.8†	80
Private:							
Postoperative	111	74	39	26	150		
PO* and return	26	45.6	31	54.4	57		
No surgery							
Clinic:							
Postoperative	23	76.7	7	23.3	30		
PO* and return	5	55.6	4	44.4	9		
No surgery							
Private and clinic:							
Postoperative	134	74.4	46	25.6	180		
PO* and return	31	47	35	53	66		
No surgery							
Total	165	67.1	81	32.9	246	52.3†	470

* Postoperative   † Of total seen who had surgery

CHART E—NODULES

	Patients Seen	Evaluation Only	%	Entered Therapy	%	Inconclusive	%	Completed Therapy	%
Private	211	54	25.6	157	74.4	6	3.8	151	96.2
Clinic	43	10	23.3	33	76.7	6	18.2	27	81.8
Private:									
Postoperative	64	11	17.2	53	82.8	3	5.7	50	94.3
PO* and return	24	6	25	18	75			18	100
No surgery	123	37	30.1	86	69.9	3	3.5	83	96.5
Clinic:									
Postoperative	20	4	20	16	80	3	18.75	13	81.25
PO* and return	5	1	20	4	80	2	50	2	50
No surgery	18	5	27.8	13	72.2	1	7.7	12	92.3
Private and clinic:									
Postoperative	84	15	17.9	69	82.1	6	8.7	63	91.3
PO* and return	29	7	24.1	22	75.9	2	9.1	20	90.9
No surgery	141	42	29.8	99	70.2	4	4	95	96
Total	254	64	25.2	190	74.8	12	6.3	178	93.7

* Postoperative

CHART E (Continued)—NODULES

	Long-term Therapy						Short-term Therapy					
	Excel.	%	Good	%	Fair	%	Excel.	%	Good	%	Fair	%
Private	37	24.5	5	3.3	2	1.3	71	47.0	19	12.6	17	11.3
Clinic	4	14.8					13	48.2	5	18.5	5	18.5
Private:												
Postoperative	7	14	2	4	1		28	48	7	14	9	18
PO* and return	8	44.4			1	5.6	7	38.91	2	11.1		
No surgery	22	26.5	3	3.6			40	48.2	10	12.1	8	9.6
Clinic:												
Postoperative	1	7.7					6	46.2	2	15.4	4	30.8
PO* and return	1	50									1	50
No surgery	2	16.7					7	58.3	3	25		
Private and clinic:												
Postoperative	8	12.7	2	3.2	1	1.6	30	47.6	9	14.3	13	20.6
PO* and return	9	45			1	5	7	35	2	10	1	5
No surgery	24	25.3	3	3.2			47	49.5	13	13.7	8	8.4
Total	41	23	5	2.8	2	1.1	84	47.2	24	13.5	22	12.4

* Postoperative

CHART E (Continued)—NODULES

| | Therapy Length Totals | | | | Therapy Results Totals | | | | | |
	Long-term	%	Short-term	%	Excel.	%	Good	%	Fair	%
Private	44	29.1	107	70.9	108	71.5	24	15.9	19	12.6
Clinic	4	14.8	23	85.2	17	63	5	18.5	5	18.5
Private:										
Postoperative	10	20	40	80	31	62	9	18	10	20
PO* and return ..	9	50	9	50	15	83.3	2	11.1	1	5.6
No surgery	25	30.1	58	69.9	62	74.7	13	15.7	8	9.6
Clinic:										
Postoperative	1	7.7	12	92.3	7	53.8	2	15.4	4	30.8
PO* and return ..	1	50	1	50	1	50			1	50
No surgery	2	16.7	10	83.3	9	75	3	25		
Private and clinic:										
Postoperative	11	17.5	52	82.5	38	60.3	11	17.5	14	22.2
PO* and return ..	10	50	10	50	16	80	2	10	2	10
No surgery	27	28.4	68	71.6	71	74.7	16	16.8	8	8.4
Total	48	27	130	73	125	70.2	29	16.3	24	13.5

* Postoperative

Modern Techniques of Vocal Rehabilitation

CHART E (Continued)—NODULES

	Number of Surgeries				Total Patients Having Surgery		Total Patients Seen
	1	%	2+	%		%	
Private	67	76.1	21	23.9	88	41.7†	211
Clinic	20	80	5	20	25	58.1†	43
Private:							
Postoperative	51	79.7	13	20.3	64		
PO* and return	16	66.7	8	33.3	24		
No surgery							
Clinic:							
Postoperative	16	80	4	20	20		
PO* and return	4	80	1	20	5		
No surgery							
Private and clinic:							
Postoperative	67	79.8	17	20.2	84		
PO* and return	20	69	9	31	29		
No surgery							
Total	87	77	26	23	113	44.5†	254

* Postoperative   † Of total seen who had surgery

CHART F—POLYPS

	Patients Seen	Evaluation Only	%	Entered Therapy	%	Inconclusive	%	Completed Therapy	%
Private	61	15	24.6	46	75.4	3	6.5	43	93.5
Clinic	7	2	28.6	5	71.4	2	40	3	60
Private:									
Postoperative	35	10	28.6	25	71.4	1	4	24	96
PO* and return	13	3	23.1	10	76.9	1	10	9	90
No surgery	13	2	15.4	11	84.6	1	9.1	10	90.9
Clinic:									
Postoperative	4	1	25	3	75			1	33.3
PO* and return	3	1	33.3	2	66.7	2	66.7	2	100
No surgery									
Private and clinic:									
Postoperative	39	11	28.2	28	71.8	3	10.7	25	89.3
PO* and return	16	4	25	12	75	1	8.3	11	91.7
No surgery	13	2	15.4	11	84.6	1	9.1	10	90.9
Total	68	17	25	51	75	5	9.8	46	90.2

* Postoperative

CHART F (Continued)—POLYPS

	Long-term Therapy						Short-term Therapy					
	Excel.	%	Good	%	Fair	%	Excel.	%	Good	%	Fair	%
Private	8	18.6	1	2.3			17	39.5	8	18.6	9	20.9
Clinic							2	66.7			1	33.3
Private:												
Postoperative	7	29.2	1	4.2			8	33.3	5	20.8	3	12.5
PO* and return	1	11.1					3	33.3	1	11.1	4	44.4
No surgery							6	60	2	20	2	20
Clinic:												
Postoperative							2	100			1	100
PO* and return												
No surgery												
Private and clinic:												
Postoperative	7	28	1	4			8	32	5	20	4	16
PO* and return	1	9.1					5	45.5	1	9.1	4	36.4
No surgery							6	60	2	20	2	20
Total	8	17.4	1	2.2			19	41.3	8	17.4	10	21.7

* Postoperative

CHART F (Continued)—POLYPS

| | Therapy Length Totals | | | | Excel. | | Therapy Results Totals | | | |
| | Long-term | | Short-term | | | | Good | | Fair | |
		%		%		%		%		%
Private	9	20.9	34	79.1	25	58.1	9	20.9	9	20.9
Clinic			3	100	2	66.7			1	33.3
Private:										
Postoperative ...	8	33.3	16	66.7	15	62.5	6	25	3	12.5
PO* and return ..	1	11.1	8	88.9	4	44.4	1	11.1	4	44.4
No surgery			10	100	6	60	2	20	2	20
Clinic:										
Postoperative ...			1	100					1	100
PO* and return ..			2	100	2	100				
No surgery										
Private and clinic:										
Postoperative ...	8	32	17	68	15	60	6	24	4	16
PO* and return ..	1	9.1	10	90.9	6	54.5	1	9.1	4	36.4
No surgery			10	100	6	60	2	20	2	20
Total	9	19.6	37	80.4	27	58.7	9	19.6	10	21.7

* Postoperative

CHART F *(Continued)*—POLYPS

	Number of Surgeries				Total Patients Having Surgery		Total Patients Seen
	1	%	2+	%		%	
Private	26	54.2	22	45.8	48	78.7†	61
Clinic	3	42.8	4	57.1	7	100†	7
Private:							
Postoperative	22	62.9	13	37.1	35		
PO* and return	4	30.8	9	69.2	13		
No surgery							
Clinic:							
Postoperative	3	75	1	25	4		
PO* and return			3	100	3		
No surgery							
Private and clinic:							
Postoperative	25	64.1	14	35.9	39		
PO* and return	4	25	12	75	16		
No surgery							
Total	29	52.7	26	47.3	55	80.9†	68

* Postoperative   † Of total seen who had surgery

CHART G—POLYPOID DEGENERATION

	Patients Seen	Evaluation Only	%	Entered Therapy	%	Inconclusive	%	Completed Therapy	%
Private	48	15	31.25	33	68.75	3	9.1	30	90.9
Clinic	15	8	53.3	7	46.7	2	28.6	5	71.4
Private:									
Postoperative	39	11	28.2	28	71.8	3	10.7	25	89.3
PO* and return	3	2	66.7	1	33.3			1	100
No surgery	6	2	33.3	4	66.7			4	100
Clinic:									
Postoperative	5	3	60	2	40			2	40
PO* and return									
No surgery	10	5	50	5	50	2	40	3	60
Private and clinic:									
Postoperative	44	14	31.8	30	68.2	3	10	27	90
PO* and return	3	2	66.7	1	33.3			1	100
No surgery	16	7	43.75	9	56.25	2	22.2	7	77.8
Total	63	23	36.5	40	63.5	5	12.5	35	87.5

* Postoperative

CHART G (*Continued*)—POLYPOID DEGENERATION

| | Long-term Therapy | | | | | | Short-term Therapy | | | | | |
	Excel.	%	Good	%	Fair	%	Excel.	%	Good	%	Fair	%
Private	6	20	1	3.3			16	53.3	5	16.7	2	6.7
Clinic	1	20							2	40	2	40
Private:												
Postoperative	6	24	1	4			12	48	4	16	2	8
PO* and return							1	100				
No surgery							3	75	1	25		
Clinic:												
Postoperative	1	50									1	50
PO* and return												
No surgery									2	66.7	1	33.3
Private and clinic:												
Postoperative	7	25.9	1	3.7			12	44.4	4	14.8	3	11.1
PO* and return							1	100				
No surgery							3	42.9	3	42.9	1	14.3
Total	7	20	1	2.9			16	45.7	7	20	4	11.4

* Postoperative

CHART G (Continued)—POLYPOID DEGENERATION

| | Therapy Length Totals | | | | Excel. | | Therapy Results Totals | | | |
	Long-term	%	Short-term	%		%	Good	%	Fair	%
Private	7	23.3	23	76.7	22	73.3	6	20	2	6.7
Clinic	1	20	4	80	1	20	2	40	2	40
Private:										
Postoperative	7	28	18	72	18	72	5	20	2	8
PO* and return			1	100	1	100				
No surgery			4	100	3	75	1	25		
Clinic:										
Postoperative	1	50	1	50	1	50			1	50
PO* and return										
No surgery			3	100			2	66.7	1	33.3
Private and clinic:										
Postoperative	8	29.6	19	70.4	19	70.4	5	18.5	3	11.1
PO* and return			1	100	1	100				
No surgery			7	100	3	42.9	3	42.9	1	14.3
Total	8	22.9	27	77.1	23	65.7	8	22.9	4	11.4

* Postoperative

CHART G (*Continued*)—POLYPOID DEGENERATION

	Number of Surgeries				Total Patients Having Surgery		Total Patients Seen
	1	%	2+	%		%	
Private	29	69	13	31	42	87.5†	48
Clinic	3	60	2	40	5	33.3†	15
Private:							
Postoperative	28	71.8	11	28.2	39		
PO* and return	1	33.3	2	66.7	3		
No surgery							
Clinic:							
Postoperative	3	60	2	40	5		
PO* and return							
No surgery							
Private and Clinic:							
Postoperative	31	70.5	13	29.5	44		
PO* and return	1	33.3	2	66.7	3		
No surgery							
Total	32	68.1	15	31.9	47	74.6†	63

* Postoperative   † Of total seen who had surgery

CHART H—CONTACT ULCERS

	Patients Seen	Evaluation Only	%	Entered Therapy	%	Inconclusive	%	Completed Therapy	%
Private	70	17	24.3	53	75.7	3	5.7	50	94.3
Clinic	15	7	46.7	8	53.3	2	25	6	75
Private:									
Postoperative	12	4	33.3	8	66.7			8	100
PO* and return	17	4	23.5	13	76.5	2	15.4	11	84.6
No surgery	41	9	22	32	78	1	3.1	31	96.9
Clinic:									
Postoperative	1	1	100						
PO* and return	1			1	100			1	100
No surgery	13	6	46.2	7	53.8	2	28.6	5	71.4
Private and clinic:									
Postoperative	13	5	38.5	8	61.5			8	100
PO* and return	18	4	22.2	14	77.8	2	14.3	12	85.7
No surgery	54	15	27.8	39	72.7	3	7.7	36	92.3
Total	85	24	28.2	61	71.8	5	8.2	56	91.8

* Postoperative

CHART H *(Continued)*—CONTACT ULCERS

| | Long-term Therapy | | | | | | Short-term Therapy | | | | | |
	Excel.	%	Good	%	Fair	%	Excel.	%	Good	%	Fair	%
Private	22	44	1	2			24	48	1	2	2	4
Clinic	2	33.3					1	16.7	3	50	2	
Private:												
Postoperative	2	25					6	75				
PO* and return	8	72.7					3	27.3				
No surgery	12	38.7	1	3.2			15	48.4	1	3.2	2	6.5
Clinic:												
Postoperative	1	100										
PO* and return	1	20					1	20	3	60		
No surgery												
Private and clinic:												
Postoperative	2	25					6	75				
PO* and return	9	75					3	25				
No surgery	13	36.1	1	2.8			16	44.4	4	11.1	2	5.6
Total	24	42.9	1	1.8			25	44.6	4	7.1	2	3.6

* Postoperative

CHART H (Continued)—CONTACT ULCERS

| | Therapy Length Totals | | | | Therapy Results Totals | | | | | |
	Long-term	%	Short-term	%	Excel.	%	Good	%	Fair	%
Private	23	46	27	54	46	92	2	4	2	4
Clinic	2	33.3	4	66.7	3	50	3	50		
Private:										
Postoperative	2	25	6	75	8	100				
PO* and return ..	8	72.7	3	27.3	11	100				
No surgery	13	41.9	18	58.1	27	87.1	2	6.5	2	6.5
Clinic:										
Postoperative	1	100			1	100				
PO* and return ..	1	20	4	80	2	40	3	60		
Private and clinic:										
Postoperative	2	25	6	75	8	100				
PO* and return ..	9	75	3	25	12	100				
No surgery	14	38.9	22	61.1	29	80.6	5	13.9	2	5.6
Total	25	44.6	31	55.4	49	87.5	5	8.9	2	3.6

* Postoperative

CHART H (*Continued*)—CONTACT ULCERS

	Number of Surgeries				Total Patients Having Surgery		Total Patients Seen
	1	%	2+	%		%	
Private	15	51.7	14	48.3	29	41.4†	70
Clinic	2	100			2	13.3†	15
Private:							
Postoperative	10	83.3	2	16.7	12		
PO* and return	5	29.4	12	70.6	17		
No surgery							
Clinic:							
Postoperative	1	100			1		
PO* and return	1	100			1		
No surgery							
Private and clinic:							
Postoperative	11	84.6	2	15.4	13		
PO* and return	6	33.3	12	66.7	18		
No surgery							
Total	17	54.8	14	45.2	31	36.5†	85

* Postoperative   † Of total seen who had surgery

CHART I

FOLLOW-UP RESULTS
COMPARISON OF THERAPIST'S AND PATIENT'S
FOLLOW-UP EVALUATION OF VOICE

Therapist	Number of Patients	%	Patient
Excellent	81	80.2	Excellent
Excellent	3	3.0	Good
Excellent			Fair
Good	12	11.9	Good
Good	3	3.0	Excellent
Good			Fair
Fair			Fair
Fair			Good
Fair	2	2.0	Excellent
Total	101		

Agreement between therapist and patient 93 or 92.1%.
Patient's self-rating higher 5 or 5%.
Patient's self-rating lower 3 or 3%.

CHART J

FOLLOW-UP RESULTS
LENGTH OF TIME BETWEEN COMPLETION OF
THERAPY AND FOLLOW-UP

Years	Number of Patients
0 to ½ yr.	10
½ to 1 yr.	40
1 to 1½ yrs.	54
1½ to 2 yrs.	17
2 to 3 yrs.	47
3 to 4 yrs.	37
4 to 5 yrs.	18
5 to 6 yrs.	14
6 to 7 yrs.	5
7 to 8 yrs.	2
10 yrs.	1
Total patients	245

The length of time from the completion of therapy to the follow-up evaluation ranged from ½ year to 10 years. The average length of time from the completion of therapy to the follow-up evaluation was approximately 2 years 7 months.

CHART K

FOLLOW-UP RESULTS
NUMBER OF PATIENTS IN FOLLOW-UP AS
GROUPED BY DYSPHONIAS

Functional Dysphonias

Functional misphonia	95
Falsetto	4
Ventricular phonation	1
Hysterical aphonia	3
Hysterical dysphonia	1
Functional aphonia	4
Spastic dysphonia	3
Incipient spastic dysphonia	5
Nasality (functional)	3
Bowed vocal folds (functional)	10
	129

Organic Dysphonias

Nodules	51
Polyps	14
Polypoid degeneration	3
Contact ulcers	24
Papillomata	2
Leukoplakia	4
Keratosis	1
Nasality (organic)	0
Bowed vocal folds (organic)	1
Paralytic dysphonia	7
Parkinson's disease	0
Neurological (other)	1
Partial cordectomy	1
Complete cordectomy	0
Hemilaryngectomy	1
Laryngectomy	6
	116

CHART L

FOLLOW-UP RESULTS
COMPLETION OF THERAPY RESULTS
COMPARED TO FOLLOW-UP RESULTS

Completion of Therapy	Number of Patients	%	Follow-up
Excellent	131	53.5	Excellent
Excellent	73	29.8	Good
Excellent	5	2.0	Fair
Good	18	7.4	Good
Good	8	3.3	Excellent
Good	6	2.4	Fair
Fair	1	.4	Fair
Fair	1	.4	Good
Fair	2	.8	Excellent
Total	245		

Patients retained vocal recovery or improved 233 or 95.1% (Follow-up good or excellent).

Patients remained fair or regressed 12 or 4.9%.

BIBLIOGRAPHY

Adler, S.: Some techniques for treating the hypernasal voice. *J Speech Hear Disord*, 25:300-302, 1960.

Anderson, V. A.: Speech needs and abilities of prospective teachers. *Q J Speech*, 30:221-225, 1944.

Anderson, V. A.: *Training the Speaking Voice*. 2nd ed. New York, Oxford Univ., 1961.

Arnold, G. E.: Spastic dysphonia: I. Changing interpretations of a persistent affliction. *Logos*, 2:3-14, 1959.

Arnold, G. E.: Vocal rehabilitation of paralytic dysphonia. VII. Paralysis of the superior laryngeal nerve. *Arch Otolaryngol*, 75:549-570, 1962a.

Arnold, G. E.: Vocal rehabilitation of paralytic dysphonia. VIII. Phoniatric methods of vocal compensation. *Arch Otolaryngol*, 76:76-83, 1962b.

Arnold, G. E.: Vocal rehabilitation of paralytic dysphonia. IX. Technique of intracordal injection. *Arch Otolaryngol*, 76:358-368, 1962c.

Arnold, G. E.: Vocal nodules and polyps: Laryngeal tissue reaction to habitual hyperkinetic dysphonia. *J Speech Hear Disord*, 27:205-217, 1962d.

Arnold, G. E.: Vocal rehabilitation of paralytic dysphonia. X. Functional results of intrachordal injection. *Arch Otolaryngol*, 78:179-186, 1963a.

Arnold, G. E.: Vocal nodules. *N Y State J Med*, 63:3096-3098, 1963b.

Arnold, G. E.: Advances in laryngeal physiology and their clinical application. *Eye, Ear, Nose, Throat Mon*, 45:78-84, 1966.

Arnold, G. E. and Pinto, S.: Ventricular dysphonia: New interpretation of an old observation. *Laryngoscope*, 70:1608-1627, 1960.

Aronson, A. E.: Speech pathology and symptom therapy in the interdisciplinary treatment of psychogenic aphonia. *J Speech Hear Disord*, 34:321-341, 1969.

Aronson, A. E., Peterson, H. W. Jr., and Litin, E. M.: Voice symptomatology in functional dysphonia and aphonia. *J Speech Hear Disord*, 29:367-380, 1964.

Aronson, A. E., Peterson, H. W. Jr., and Litin, E. M.: Psychiatric symptomatology in functional dysphonia and aphonia. *J Speech Hear Disord*, 31:115-127, 1966.

Aronson, A. E., Brown, J. R., Litin, E. M., and Pearson, J. S.: Spastic dysphonia. I. Voice, neurologic, and psychiatric aspects. *J Speech Hear Disord*, 33:203-218, 1968a.

Aronson, A. E., Brown, J. R., Litin, E. M., and Pearson, J. S.: Spastic dysphonia. II. Comparison with essential (voice) tremor and other neurologic and psychogenic dysphonias. *J Speech Hear Disord*, 33:219-231, 1968b.

Ash, J. E. and Schwartz, L.: The laryngeal (vocal cord) node, *Trans Am Acad Ophthalmol Otolaryngol*, 48:323-332, 1944.

Baker, D. C.: Contact ulcers of the larynx. *Laryngoscope*, 64:73-78, 1954.

Baker, D. C.: Laryngeal problems in singers. *Laryngoscope*, 72:902-908, 1962.

Baker, D. C.: Polypoid vocal cord. *N Y State J Med*, 63:3098-3099, 1963.

Baker, D. C.: Benign tumors of the larynx. *Trans Pac Coast Otoophthalmol Soc*, 49:293-299, 1965.

Bangs, J. L. and Freidinger, A.: Diagnosis and treatment of a case of hysterical aphonia in a thirteen year old girl. *J Speech Hear Disord*, 14:312-317, 1949.

Bangs, J. L. and Freidinger, A.: A case of hysterical dysphonia in an adult. *J Speech Hear Disord*, 15:316-323, 1950.

Baron, S. H. and Kohlmoos, H. W.: Laryngeal sequelae of endotracheal anesthesia. *Ann Otol*, 60:767-792, 1951.

Barton, R. T.: The whispering syndrome of hysterical dysphonia. *Ann Otol*, 69:156-164, 1960.

Bauer, H.: Die Beeinflussung der weiblichen Stimme durch androgene Hormone. (Influencing the feminine voice with androgenous hormones.) *Folia Phoniatr*, 15:264-268, 1963.

Bauer, H.: Stimm- und Sprachstörungen als Nebenwirkungen von Arzneimitteln. *Internat Assoc Logopedics Phoniatr*, 14:239-246, 1968.

Baynes, R.: An incidence study of chronic hoarseness among children. *J Speech Hear Disord*, 31:172-175, 1966.

Bergström, J.: Post-intubation granuloma of the larynx. *Acta Otolaryngol*, 57:113-118, 1964.

Bergström, J., Moberg, A., and Orell, S. R.: On the pathogenesis of laryngeal injuries following prolonged intubation. *Acta Otolaryngol*, 55:342-346, 1962.

Bicknell, J. M., Greenhouse, A. H., and Pesch, R. N.: Spastic dysphonia. *J Neurol Neurosurg Psychiatry*, 31:158-161, 1968.

Bjork, H. and Weber, C.: Papilloma of the larynx. *Acta Otolaryngol*, 46:499-516, 1956.

Bloch, E. L. and Goodstein, L. D.: Functional speech disorders and personality: A decade of research. *J Speech Hear Disord*, 36:295-314, 1971.

Bloch, P.: Goals and limits of vocal analysis. *Logos*, 2:111-118, 1959.

Bloch, P.: Some psychological and neuro-psychiatrical aspects of voice and speech therapy. *Internat Assoc Logopedics Phoniatr*, 12:130-134, 1962.

Bloch, P.: Dysphonies de réfuge. (Dysphonias as refuges.) *J Fr Otorhinolaryngol*, 13:309-313, 1964.

Bloch, P.: Neuro-psychiatric aspects of spastic dysphonia. *Folia Phoniatr*, 17:301-364, 1965.

Boedts, D., Roels, H., and Kluyskens, P.: Laryngeal tissue responses to teflon. *Arch Otolaryngol*, 86:562-567, 1967.

Boland, J. L.: Voice therapy for hoarse voice. *J Okla State Med Assoc,* 46:109-113, 1953.

Boone, D. R.: Treatment of functional aphonia in a child and an adult. *J Speech Hear Disord,* 31:69-74, 1966.

Boone, D. R.: *The Voice and Voice Therapy.* Englewood Cliffs, Prentice-Hall, 1971.

Brewer, D. W. and Briess, F. B.: Voice problems. *Med Times,* 88:461-464, 1960a.

Brewer, D. W. and Briess, F. B.: Industrial noise: Laryngeal considerations. *N Y State J Med,* 60:1737-1740, 1960b.

Briess, F. B.: Voice therapy; Part I. Identification of specific laryngeal muscle dysfunction by voice testing. *Arch Otolaryngol,* 66:375-381, 1957.

Brodnitz, F. S.: *Keep Your Voice Healthy.* New York, Harper and Brothers, 1953.

Brodnitz, F. S.: Voice problems of the actor and singer. *J Speech Hear Disord,* 19:322-326, 1954.

Brodnitz, F. S.: Vocal rehabilitation in benign lesions of the vocal cords. *J Speech Hear Disord,* 23:112-117, 1958.

Brodnitz, F. S.: The holistic study of the voice. *Q J Speech,* 48:280-284, 1962.

Brodnitz, F. S.: Functional disorders of the voice. In Levin, N. M. (Ed.): *Voice and Speech Disorders: Medical Aspects.* Springfield, Thomas, 1962.

Brodnitz, F. S.: Goals, results, and limitations of vocal rehabilitation. *Arch Otolaryngol,* 77:148-156, 1963.

Brodnitz, F. S.: Rehabilitation of the human voice. *Bull New York Acad Med,* 42:231-240, 1966a.

Brodnitz, F. S.: Training of students in the management of disorders of voice. *ASHA,* 8:270-273, 1966b.

Brodnitz, F. S.: Functional aphonia. *Ann Otol,* 78:1244-1253, 1969.

Brodnitz, F. S.: Hormones and the human voice. *Bull N Y Acad Med,* 47:183-191, 1971.

Bryngelson, B.: The functional falsetto voice. *Speech Teacher,* 3:127-128, 1954.

Calvet, J. and Coll, J.: Trois cas de masculinisation de la voix par pellets de testosterone. (Three cases of masculinization of the voice through testosterone pills.) *J Franc Otorhinolaryngol,* 13:287-290, 1964.

Canter, G. J.: Speech characteristics of patients with Parkinson's disease: I. Intensity, pitch, and duration. *J Speech Hear Disord,* 28:221-229, 1963.

Carrell, J.: Functional training as an adjunct in the management of dysphonia. *Trans Pacific Coast Oto-Ophth Soc,* 44:257-261, 1963.

Cavanaugh, J. A.: Benign neoplasms of larynx. *Illinois Med J,* 43:59-64, 1923.

Clerf, L. H.: Treatment of chronic laryngitis simplex. *Amer Acad Ophth Otolaryngol*, 42:384-391, 1937.

Clerf, L. H.: Laryngeal disease. *Proc First Institute on Voice Pathology*, Cleveland, Cleveland Hearing and Speech Center, 1952, pp. 3-7, 15-18.

Cooper, M.: *Vocal Manifestations of Laryngeal Papillomatosis*. Unpublished Ph.D. Dissertation. University of California at Los Angeles, 1964.

Cooper, M.: The habitual pitch of normal speakers throughout the day. Unpublished study, University of California at Los Angeles Medical Center, 1965.

Cooper, M.: Vocal suicide in the legal profession. *Bar Bull*, 43:453-456, 1968.

Cooper, M.: In consultation. *Med Trib*, 10:13, 1969a.

Cooper, M.: Vocal suicide in the theatrical profession. *Screen Actor*, 11:8-9, 1969b.

Cooper, M.: The pitch level of television commercials and the vocal image. Unpublished study, 1969c.

Cooper, M.: Rehabilitation of paralytic dysphonia. *Calif Med*, 112:18-20, 1970a.

Cooper, M.: Vocal rehabilitation—current opinion. *Med Trib*, 11:11, 1970b.

Cooper, M.: Vocal suicide in singers. *Bull Nat Assoc Teachers Singing*, 26:7-10, 31, 1970c.

Cooper, M.: Teacher, save that voice! *Grade Teacher*, 87:71-72, 74, 76, 1970d.

Cooper, M.: Speech disorders and problems. *Ped News*, 4:27, 48, 1970e.

Cooper, M.: Vocal suicide in teachers. *Peabody J Ed*, 47:334-337, 1970f.

Cooper, M.: Voice problems of the geriatric patient. *Geriatrics*, 25:107-110, 1970g.

Cooper, M.: Vocal suicide among theologians. *Your Church*, 3:16-21, 1970h.

Cooper, M.: Vocal suicide of the speaking voice in singers. *Music Ed J*, 57:52-54, 1970i.

Cooper, M.: A broadcaster's artistic voice. *Quill*, 58:19, 1970j.

Cooper, M.: Voice therapy for teachers. *Education*, 91:142-146, 1970k.

Cooper, M.: Vocal suicide in newscasters and announcers: The "impressive" voice. *Radio-TV News Dir Assoc Bull*, 21, 1970l.

Cooper, M.: Rehabilitation of paralytic dysphonia. *Eye Ear Nose Throat Mon*, 49:532-535, 1970m.

Cooper, M.: The vocal image and vocal suicide. *Voices: The Art and Science of Psychotherapy*, 6:26-28, 1970n.

Cooper, M.: Papillomata of the vocal folds: I. Review of the literature II. A program of vocal rehabilitation. *J Speech Hear Disord*, 36:51-60, 1971a.

Cooper, M.: Speech disorders and problems. *Ped News*, 5:48-49, 1971b.

Cooper, M.: Modern techniques of vocal rehabilitation for functional and organic dysphonias. In Travis, Lee E. (Ed.): *Handbook of Speech Pathology and Audiology*. New York, Appleton-Century-Crofts, 1971c.

Cooper, M.: Spectrographic analysis of fundamental frequency and voice quality before and after vocal rehabilitation. Unpublished study, 1972.

Cooper, M. and Nahum, A. M.: Vocal rehabilitation for contact ulcer of the larynx. *Arch Otolaryngol*, 85:41-46, 1967.

Cooper, M. and Yanagihara, N.: A study of basal pitch level variations found in the normal speaking voices of males and females. *J Commun Dis*, 3:261-266, 1971.

Corbetta, L. and Felletti, V.: Osservazioni cliniche ed ipotesi patogenetiche sul granuloma laringeo da intubazione. (Clinical observations and hypothesis on the pathogenesis of laryngeal granuloma following intubation.) *Arch Ital Otol*, 72:513-523, 1961.

Cornut, G. and Cornut, C.: Abaissement pathologique du registre vocal chez la femme. (Pathological lowering of the vocal register in women.) *J Franc Otorhinolaryngol*, 14:59-69, 1965.

Cornut, G. and Pierucci, B.: Contribution à l'étude de la paralysie récurrentielle du point de vue phoniatrique. (Contribution to the study of recurrent paralysis from the phoniatric point of view.) *J Franc Otorhinolaryngol*, 17:665-672, 1968.

Cornut, G. and Rebattu, J. P.: Appréciation médico-légale des séquelles des traumatismes laryngées. (Medico-legal estimation of the sequelae of laryngeal traumatisms.) *J Franc Otorhinolaryngol*, 18:533-540, 1969.

Cornut, G. and Venet, C.: Les dysphonies chroniques de l'enfant d'âge scolaire. (Chronic dysphonias of the school-age child.) *J Franc Otorhinolaryngol*, 15:837-852, 1966.

Cracovaner, A. J.: Premalignant diseases of the larynx. *Pacific Med Surg*, 73:176-180, 1965.

Cunning, D. S.: Benign neoplasms of the larynx. *New York J Med*, 34:56-58, 1934.

Cunning, D. S.: Diagnosis and treatment of laryngeal tumors. *JAMA* 142:73-77, 1950.

Curry, E. T.: Hoarseness and voice change in male adolescents. *J Speech Hear Disord*, 14:23-25, 1949.

Damsté, P. H.: Virilization of the voice due to anabolic steroids. *Folia Phoniatr*, 16:10-18, 1964.

Damsté, P. H.: Voice change in adult women caused by virilizing agents. *J Speech Hear Disord*, 32:126-132, 1967.

Darley, F. L.: Clinical training for full-time clinical service: A neglected obligation. *ASHA*, 11:143-148, 1969.

Davis, D. S. and Boone, D. R.: Pitch discrimination and tonal memory abilities in adult voice patients. *J Speech Hear Res*, 10:811-815, 1967.

Dekelboum, A.: Papillomas of the larynx. *Arch Otolaryngol*, 81:390-397, 1965.

Diehl, C., and McDonald, E. T.: Effect of voice quality on communication. *J Speech Hear Disord*, 21:233-237, 1956.

Doehler, M.: *Esophageal Speech*. Boston, American Cancer Society, 1956.

Douglas, T. E.: Hoarseness. *Northwest Med*, 49:383-385, 1950.

Duncan, M. H.: Personality adjustment techniques in voice therapy. *J Speech Disord*, 12:161-167, 1947.

Eisenson, J.: *The Improvement of Voice and Diction*. 2nd ed. New York, Macmillan Co., 1965.

Eisenson, J., Kastein, S., and Schneiderman, N.: An investigation into the ability of voice defectives to discriminate among differences in pitch and loudness. *J Speech Hear Disord*, 23:577-582, 1958.

El-Mofti, A.: Laryngeal polypoid growths following endotracheal anaesthesia. *J Laryngol*, 63:759-761, 1949.

Fairbanks, G.: *Voice and Articulation Drillbook*. 2nd ed. New York, Harper & Brothers, 1960.

Farrior, J. B.: Contact ulcer of the larynx developing after intratracheal anesthesia. *Arch Otolaryngol*, 36:238-239, 1942.

Ferguson, C. F. and Scott, H. W.: Papillomatosis of the larynx in childhood. *New Eng J Med*, 230:477-482, 1944.

Ferguson, G. B.: Organic lesions of the larynx produced by mis-use of the voice. *Laryngoscope*, 65:327-336, 1955.

Fisher, H. B. and Logemann, J. A.: Objective evaluation of therapy for vocal nodules: A case report. *J Speech Hear Disord*, 35:277-285, 1970.

Fitz-Hugh, G. S., Smith, D. E., and Chiong, A. T.: Pathology of three hundred clinically benign lesions of the vocal cords. *Trans Am Laryngol Rhino Otol Soc*, 61:476-496, 1958.

Flatau, T.: *Die Funktionelle Stimmsahwacche (Phoniasthenie)*. Berlin, Buerkner, 1906.

Flower, R. M.: Voice training in the management of dysphonia. *Laryngoscope*, 69:940-946, 1959.

Fox, D. R.: Spastic dysphonia: A case presentation. *J Speech Hear Disord*, 34:275-279, 1969.

Frable, M. A. S.: Hoarseness, a symptom of premenstrual tension. *Arch Otolaryngol*, 75:66-68, 1962.

Fred, H. L.: Hoarseness due to phonation by the false vocal cords. *Arch Int Med*, 110:472-475, 1962.

Freud, E. D.: Functions and dysfunctions of the ventricular folds. *J Speech Hear Disord*, 27:334-340, 1962.

Frick, J. V.: Incidence of voice defects among school-age speech defective children. *Pennsylvania Speech Ann*, 17:61-62, 1960.

Friedberg, S. A. and Segall, W. H.: The pathologic anatomy of polyps of the larynx. *Ann Otol*, 50:783-789, 1941.

Froeschels, E.: Hygiene of the voice. *Arch Otolaryngol*, 38:122-130, 1943.

Froeschels, E.: Experiences of a bloodless treatment for recurrens—paralysis. *J Laryngol*, 59:347-358, 1944.

Froeschels, E.: Should the speech therapist be a voice therapist? *J Speech Hear Disord*, 13:346-350, 1948.

Froeschels, E., Kastein, S., and Weiss, D. A.: A method of therapy for paralytic conditions of the mechanisms of phonation, respiration, and glutination. *J Speech Hear Disord*, 20:365-370, 1955.

Gabriel, C. E. and Jones, D. G.: The importance of chronic laryngitis. *J Laryngol*, 74:349-357, 1960.

Gardner, W. H.: Executive's dysphonia: A study of 49 patients. *Cleveland Clin Quart*, 25:177-186, 1958.

Gildston, P. and Gildston, H.: The problem of validity in determining optimum pitch levels. *Internat Assoc Logopedics Phoniatr*, 14:124-126, 1968.

Glasgow, G.: The effects of nasality on oral communication. *Q J Speech*, 30:337-342, 1944.

Goldman, D.: Management of psychosomatic problems in young adults. *Psychiat Dig*, 28:33-37; 39; 42-43; 46, 1967.

Goldman, J. L., and Salmon, U.: The effect of androgen therapy on the voice and vocal cords of adult women. *Ann Otol*, 51:961-968, 1942.

Goodstein, L.: Functional speech disorders and personality: A survey of the research. *J Speech Hear Res*, 1:359-376, 1958.

Gray, G. W. (Ed.): *Studies in Experimental Phonetics, University Studies No. 27*. Baton Rouge, Louisiana St Univ Press, 1936.

Greene, M.: *The Voice and Its Disorders*. 2nd ed. London, Pitman Medical, 1964.

Greene, M.: Vocal disabilities of singers. *Proc R Soc Med*, 61:1150-1152, 1968.

Greene, M., and Watson, B. W.: The value of speech amplification in Parkinson's disease patients. *Folia Phoniatr*, 20:250-257, 1968.

Grimaud, R. and Bonneville, J.: Anabolisants de synthèse et voix. *Rev Laryngol*, 85:734-742, 1964.

Gundermann, H.: Phoniatrische Bemerkungen zur sogenannten Lehrerkrankheit. (Phoniatric notes in connection with the so-called "teachers' disease.") *Dtsch Gesundheitsw—Wes*, 18:69-72, 1963.

Gundermann, H., Weuffen, M., and Lüth, C.: Die logopädische Therapie im Rahmen der komplexen Stimmheilkur. (Logopedic therapy within the limits of the complex remedial voice training.) *Folia Phoniatr*, 18:183-196, 1966.

Guthrie, D.: The pathology of speech and voice. *Edinburgh Med J*, 47:391-405, 1940.

Hanley, T. D., and Steer, M. D.: Effect of level of distracting noise upon speaking rate, duration, and intensity. *J Speech Hear Disord*, 14:363-368, 1949.

Hanley, T. D., and Thurman, W.: *Developing Vocal Skills*. New York, Holt, Rinehart and Winston, 1962.

322 Modern Techniques of Vocal Rehabilitation

Harris, R.: Comments on a particular type of hoarseness. *Trans Am Laryngol Rhino Otol Soc,* 63:182-183, 1960.

Harrison, G. A. and Tonkin, J. P.: Some serious laryngeal complications of prolonged endotracheal intubation. *Med J. Aust,* 1:605-606, 1967.

Heaver, L.: Psychiatric observations on the personality structure of patients with habitual dysphonia. *Logos,* 1:21-26, 1958.

Heaver, L.: Spastic dysphonia: II. Psychiatric considerations. *Logos,* 2:15-24, 1959.

Heaver, L.: Spastic dysphonia. In Barbara, D. A. (Ed.): *Psychological and Psychiatric Aspects of Speech and Hearing.* Springfield, Thomas, 1960.

Heinberg, P.: *Voice Training for Speaking and Reading Aloud.* New York, Ronald Press, 1964.

Henrikson, E. H., and Irwin, J. V.: Voice recording—some findings and some problems. *J Speech Hear Disord,* 14:227-233, 1949.

Holinger, P. H., and Johnston, K. C.: Benign tumors of the larynx. *Ann Otol,* 60:496-509, 1951.

Holinger, P. H., and Johnston, K. C.: Contact ulcer of the larynx. *JAMA,* 172:511-515, 1960.

Holinger, P. H., Schild, J. A., and Maurizi, D. G.: Laryngeal papilloma: Review of etiology and therapy. *Laryngoscope,* 78:1462-1474, 1968.

Hollien, H., Moore, G. P., Wendahl, R. W., and Michel, J. F.: On the nature of vocal fry. *J Speech Hear Res,* 9:245-247, 1966.

Hollien, H., and Wendahl, R. W.: Perceptual study of vocal fry. *J Acoust Soc Am,* 43:506-509, 1968.

Holmes, F. L. D.: An experimental study of individual vocal quality. *Q J Speech,* 16:344-351, 1930.

Holmes, F. L. D.: The problem of voice placement. *Q J Speech,* 17:236-245, 1931

Hoopes, J. E., Dellon, A. L., Fabrikant, J. I., and Soliman, A. H.: Idiopathic hypernasality: Cineradiographic evaluation and etiologic considerations. *J Speech Hear Disord,* 35:44-50, 1970.

House, A.: A note on optimal vocal frequency. *J Speech Hear Res,* 2:55-60, 1959.

Huizinga, E.: Papilloma laryngis. *Ann Otol,* 66:1075-1079, 1957.

Huyck, M., and Allen, K.: Diaphragmatic action of good and poor speaking voices. *Speech Monogr,* 4:101-109, 1937.

Imre, V.: Hormonbedingte stimmstörungen und ihre behandlung. *Internat Assoc Logopedics Phoniatr,* 13:139-142, 1965.

Jackson, C.: Contact ulcer of the larynx. *Ann Otol,* 37:227-230, 1928.

Jackson, C.: Myasthenia laryngis. *Arch Otolaryngol,* 32:434-463, 1940.

Jackson, C., and Jackson, C. L.: Contact ulcer of the larynx. *Trans Sect Laryng Otol Rhino AMA,* 86:69-88, 1935a.

Jackson, C., and Jackson, C. L.: Dysphonia plicae ventricularis: Phonation with the ventricular bands. *Arch Otolaryngol,* 21:157-167, 1935b.

Jackson, C., and Jackson, C. L.: *Cancer of the Larynx.* Philadelphia, W. B. Saunders, 1939.

Jackson, C. L.: Neoplasms of the larynx, lower respiratory tract, and esophagus. In Coates, H. M., and Schenck, H. P. (Eds.): *Otolaryngology.* Hagerstown, W. F. Prior, 1960, Vol. 5.

Kallen, L. A.: What is "optimal" for the human voice? *Logos,* 2:40-48, 1959.

Kelly, H. D. B., and Craik, J. E.: Laryngeal nodes and the so-called amyloid tumour of the cords. *J Laryngol,* 66:339-358, 1952.

Kernan, J. D.: Fundamental pathology of the larynx. *Laryngoscope,* 47: 77-91, 1937.

Kleinsasser, O.: *Microlaryngoscopy and Endolaryngeal Microsurgery.* Hoffman, P. W. (Trans.) Philadelphia, W. B. Saunders, 1968.

Knower, F. H., and Emerson, M.: Indices of achievement in voice instruction. *J Speech Disord,* 11:159-163, 1946.

König, W. F.: Laryngeale Komplikationen infolge langer Verweildauer von Nährsonden. (Laryngeal complications due to feeding tubes being left in situ for long periods of time.) *Prakt Anästh,* 2:164-166, 1967.

Kürthy, S. A.: Granulomul laringian după intubatie traheală. (Laryngeal granuloma following tracheal intubation.) *Otorinolaringol ORL Ruman,* 11:235-241, 1966.

Labastida, L.: A proposito de 150 peritajes foniatricos en maestras de escuela primaria. (On the subject of 150 phoniatric surveys of primary school teachers.) *Acta Otorinolaringol Iber Am,* 12:200-203, 1961.

Ladefoged, P.: Professor of Phonetics, Department of Linguistics, University of California at Los Angeles. Personal Communication.

Laguaite, J. K., and Waldrop, W. F.: Acoustic analysis of fundamental frequency of voices before and after therapy. *Folia Phoniatr,* 16:183-192, 1964.

Legget, R. F., and Northwood, T. D.: Noise surveys of cocktail parties. *J Acoust Soc Am,* 32:16-18, 1960.

Lejska, V.: Profesionálńi poruchy hlasu u učitelů. (Occupational voice disorders of teachers.) *Pracov Lék,* 19:119-121, 1967.

Lell, W. A.: Diagnosis and direct laryngoscopic treatment of functional aphonia. *Arch Otolaryngol,* 34:141-149, 1941.

Lerman, J. W., and Duffy, R. J.: Recognition of falsetto voice quality. *Folia Phoniatr,* 22:21-27, 1970.

Levin, N. M.: Benign and malignant lesions of the larynx. In Levin, N. M. (Ed.): *Voice and Speech Disorders: Medical Aspects.* Springfield, Thomas, 1962.

Lewy, R. B.: Responses of laryngeal tissue to granular teflon in situ. *Arch Otolaryngol,* 83:355-359, 1966.

Lieberman, P.: Some acoustic measures of the fundamental periodicity of normal and pathologic larynges. *J Acoust Soc Am,* 35:344-353, 1963.

Lore, J. M.: Hoarseness in children. *Arch Otolaryngol,* 51:814-825, 1950.

Lu, A. T., Tamura, Y., and Koobs, D. H.: The pathology of laryngotracheal complications. *Arch Otolaryngol,* 74:323-332, 1961.

Luchsinger, R., and Arnold, G. E.: *Voice-Speech-Language.* Belmont, Wadsworth, 1965.

Luse, E. M.: Occupations of laryngectomees prior to surgery. *Internat Assoc Logopedics Phoniatr,* 13:191-193, 1965.

McClosky, D. B.: *Your Voice at Its Best.* Boston, Little, Brown, 1959.

McGlone, R. E., and Hollien, H.: Vocal pitch characteristics of aged women. *J Speech Hear Res,* 6:164-170, 1963.

Maier, I.: Maligne entartung bestrahlter juveniler larynxpapillome. (Malignant degeneration of juvenile papilloma of the larynx.) *Z Laryngol Rhinol Otol,* 47:862-869, 1968.

Majoros, M., Parkhill, E., and Devine, K. D.: Papilloma of the larynx in children. *Am J Surg,* 108:470-475, 1964.

Manser, R. B.: Voice problems of university students. *Am Speech Corr Assoc,* 9:90-102, 1939.

Meano, C.: *The Human Voice in Speech and Song,* Rev. ed. Khoury, A. (Trans.) Springfield, Thomas, 1967.

Michel, J. F.: Fundamental frequency investigation of vocal fry and harshness. *J Speech Hear Res,* 11:590-594, 1968.

Mitchell, H. E.: Tumors of the larynx. A review of 105 cases. *Trans Am Laryngol Rhino Otol Soc,* 46:249-268, 1943.

Moore, G. P.: Voice disorders associated with organic abnormalities. In Travis, L. E. (Ed.): *Handbook of Speech Pathology.* New York, Appleton-Century-Crofts, 1957.

Moore, G. P.: *Organic Voice Disorders.* Englewood Cliffs, Prentice-Hall, 1971.

Mosby, D. P.: Psychotherapy versus voice therapy for a child with a deviant voice, a case study. *Percept Mot Skills,* 30:887-891, 1970.

Moser, H. M., Dreher, J. J., and Adler, S.: Comparison of hyponasality, hypernasality, and normal voice quality on the intelligibility of two-digit numbers. *J Acoust Soc Am,* 27:872-874, 1955.

Moses, P. J.: Is medical phonetics an essential part of otorhinolaryngology? *Arch Otolaryngol,* 31:444-450, 1940.

Moses, P. J.: Vocal analysis. *Arch Otolaryngol,* 48:171-186, 1948.

Moses, P. J.: *The Voice of Neurosis.* New York, Grune and Stratton, 1954.

Muma, J. R., Laeder, R. L., and Webb, C. E.: Adolescent voice quality aberrations: Personality and social status. *J Speech Hear Res,* 11:576-582, 1968.

Murphy, A. T.: *Functional Voice Disorders.* Englewood Cliffs, Prentice-Hall, 1964.

Murphy, R. S.: Hoarseness. *N S Med Bull,* 46:177-179, 1967.

Myerson, M. C.: *The Human Larynx.* Springfield, Thomas, 1964.

Mysak, E. D.: Pitch and duration characteristics of older males. *J Speech Hear Res*, 2:46-54, 1959.

Nemec, J.: The motivation background of hyperkinetic dysphonia in children: A contribution to psychologic research in phoniatry. *Logos*, 4:28-31, 1961.

New, G. B., and Devine, K. D.: Contact ulcer granuloma. *Ann Otol*, 58: 548-558, 1949.

New, G. B., and Erich, J. B.: Benign tumors of the larynx: A study of seven hundred and twenty-two cases. *Arch Otolaryngol*, 28:841-910, 1938.

O'Neil, J. J., and McGee, J. A.: Management of benign laryngeal tumors in children: Preoperative, operative, and postoperative. *Ann Otol*, 71: 480-488, 1962.

Pahn, J.: Der therapeutische wert nasaliertor vokalklänge in der Behandlung funktioneller Stimmerkrankungen. (Therapy utilizing nasalized vowels in the treatment of functional dysphonia.) *Folia Phoniatr*, 16: 249-263, 1964.

Pahn, J.: Zur Entwicklung und Behandlung funktioneller Singstimmerkrankungen. (The development and treatment of functional disorders of the singing voice.) *Folia Phoniatr*, 18:117-130, 1966.

Pahn, J., and Glatz, E.: (The prophylaxis of disorders of voice production and speech in kindergarten and at school.) *Z Arztl Fortbild*, 63:351-354, 1969.

Preacher, G. M.: Contact ulcer of the larynx; I. History. *J Speech Disord*, 12:67-76, 1947a.

Peacher, G. M.: Contact ulcer of the larynx; III. Etiological factors. *J Speech Disord*, 12:177-178, 1947b.

Peacher, G. M.: Contact ulcer of the larynx; IV. A clinical study of vocal re-education. *J Speech Disord*, 12:179-190, 1947c.

Peacher, G. M.: Voice therapy for ulcers and nodules of the larynx. *Proc First Institute on Voice Pathology*. Cleveland, Cleveland Speech and Hearing Center, 1952, pp. 7-18.

Peacher, G. M.: Vocal therapy for contact ulcer of the larynx. A follow-up of seventy patients. *Laryngoscope*, 71:34-47, 1961.

Peacher, G. M.: Voice therapy. *N Y State J Med*, 63:3104-3107, 1963.

Peacher, G. M.: *How to Improve Your Speaking Voice*. New York, Frederick Fell, 1966.

Peacher, G. M., and Holinger, P.: Contact ulcer of the larynx; II. The role of vocal re-education. *Arch Otolaryngol*, 46:617-623, 1947.

Perkins, W. H.: The challenge of functional disorders of voice. In Travis, L. E. (Ed.): *Handbook of Speech Pathology*. New York, Appleton-Century-Crofts, 1957.

Pietrantoni, L., and Fior, R.: Problems of cancer of the larynx. *Acta Otolaryngol*, Suppl 142, pp. 14-16, 1958.

Pleet, L.: Private practice (Otolaryngology), Encino, California.

Powers, M. H.: The dichotomy in our profession. *J Speech Hear Disord,* 20:4-10, 1955.

Pronovost, W.: An experimental study of methods for determining natural and habitual pitch. *Speech Monogr,* 9:111-123, 1942.

Rabbett, W.: Juvenile laryngeal papillomatosis. *Ann Otol,* 74:1149-1163, 1965.

Riesman, D. with Glazer, N. and Denney, R.: *The Lonely Crowd.* New Haven, Yale Univ., 1950.

Riker, B. L.: The ability to judge pitch. *J Exp Psychol,* 36:331-346, 1946.

Robe, E., Brumlik, J., and Moore, P.: A study of spastic dysphonia. Neurologic and electroencephalographic abnormalities. *Laryngoscope,* 70: 219-245, 1960.

Rosenbaum, H. D., Alavi, S. M., and Bryant, L. R.: Pulmonary parenchymal spread of juvenile laryngeal papillomatosis. *Radiology,* 90:654-660, 1968.

Rubin, H. J.: Assistant Clinical Professor, Dept of Head and Neck Surgery, UCLA School of Medicine.

Rubin, H. J.: Intracordal injection of silicone in selected dysphonias. *Arch Otolaryngol,* 81:604-607, 1965a.

Rubin, H. J.: Pitfalls in treatment of dysphonias by intracordal injection of synthetics. *Laryngoscope,* 75:1381-1397, 1965b.

Rubin, H. J.: Histologic and high-speed photographic observations on the intracordal injection of synthetics. *Trans Am Acad Ophthalmol Otolaryngol,* 70:909-921, 1967.

Rubin, J. A.: Papilloma of the larynx. *Can Med Assoc J,* 71:572-575, 1954.

Russell, G. O.: Etiology of follicular pharyngitis, catarrhal laryngitis, so-called clergyman's throat; and singer's nodes. *J Speech Disord,* 1:113-122, 1936.

Salinger, S.: Benign tumors of the vocal cord. *Trans Am Laryngol Assoc,* 77:186-197, 1956.

Sallee, W. H.: An objective study of respiration in relation to audibility in connected speech. In Gray, G. W. (Ed.): *Studies in Experimental Phonetics, University Studies No. 27.* Baton Rouge, Louisiana St Univ Press, 1936, pp. 52-58.

Sarbin, T. R.: Role theoretical interpretation of psychological change. In Worchel, P., and Byrne, D. (Eds.): *Personality Change.* New York, Wiley, 1964.

Satou, A., and Cooper, M.: Psychiatric observation of falsetto voice. *The Voice,* 17:31-33, 35-37, 39, 41, 1968.

Schick, A.: Functional therapy in vocal disabilities. *Folia Phoniatr,* 18: 138-143, 1966.

Schoolfield, L. D.: *Better Speech and Better Reading.* Magnolia, Expression, 1951.

Senturia, B. H., and Wilson, F. B.: Otorhinolaryngic findings in children with voice deviations. *Ann Otol,* 77:1027-1041, 1968.

Shanks, J.: A short study of papilloma of the larynx. *Arch Otolaryngol,* 67: 219-221, 1958.

Shearer, W. M.: Cybernetics in the treatment of voice disorders. *J Speech Hear Disord,* 24:280-282, 1959.

Sheehan, J. G.: *Stuttering: Research and Therapy.* New York, Harper & Row, 1970.

Sherman, D., and Goodwin, F.: Pitch level and nasality. *J Speech Hear Disord,* 19:423-428, 1954.

Snidecor, J. C.: A comparative study of the pitch and duration characteristics of impromptu speaking and oral reading. *Speech Monogr,* 10:50-56, 1943.

Snidecor, J. C.: The pitch and duration characteristics of superior female speakers during oral reading. *J Speech Hear Disord,* 16:44-52, 1951.

Snidecor, J. C., and others: *Speech Rehabilitation of the Laryngectomized.* 2nd ed. Springfield, Thomas, 1968.

Stewart, J. P.: The histo-pathology of benign tumours of the larynx. *J Laryngol,* 71:718-729, 1957.

Szpunar, J.: Laryngeal papillomatosis. *Acta Otolaryngol,* 63:74-86, 1967.

Tarneaud, J.: Une laryngopathie fonctionnelle: La voix aggravée. *Folia Phoniatr,* 1:7-14, 1947.

Tarneaud, J.: The fundamental principles of vocal cultivation and therapeutics of the voice. *Logos,* 1:7-10, 1958.

Thurman, W. L.: Frequency-intensity relationships and optimal pitch level. *J Speech Hear Res,* 1:117-123, 1958.

Toomey, J. M., and Brown, B. S.: The histological response to intracordal injection of teflon paste. *Laryngoscope,* 77:110-120, 1967.

Tucker, G.: Observations on chronic inflammatory lesions of the true vocal cords. *Trans Am Acad Ophthalmol Otolaryngol,* 40:390-402, 1935.

Tucker, G.: Tumors of the true vocal cords: Malignant, benign. *Trans Sect Laryngol Otol Rhino AMA,* 88:171-177, 1937.

Ullmann, E. V.: On the aetiology of the laryngeal papilloma. *Acta Otolaryngol,* 5:317-334, 1923.

Van Deinse, J. B., Dieleman, F., and Drost, H. A.: La révalidation des troubles de la voix virilisée par des médicaments. (The rehabilitation of the voice virilized by medicines.) *Pract Otorhinolaryngol,* 28:288-293, 1966.

Van Riper, C.: *Speech Correction: Principles and Methods,* 4th ed. New York, Prentice-Hall, 1963.

Van Riper, C., and Irwin, J. V.: *Voice and Articulation.* Englewood Cliffs, Prentice-Hall, 1958.

van Thal, J. H.: Dysphonia. *Speech Path Ther,* 4:11-21, 1961.

Van Wye, B. C.: The efficient voice in speech. *Q J Speech,* 22:642-648, 1936.

Vennard, W.: An experiment to evaluate the importance of nasal resonance in singing. *Internat Assoc Logopedics Phoniatr,* 12:418-419, 1962.

Virchow, R.: *Die Cellularpathologie in ihrer Begründung auf physiologische und pathologische Gewebelehre.* Berlin, Hirschwald, 1858.

Voelker, C. H.: Phoniatry in dysphonia ventricularis. *Ann Otol,* 44:471-473, 1935.

Voelker, C. H.: Frequency of hoarseness due to phonation with the thyroarytenoid lips. Jackson's dysphonia plicae ventricularis. *Arch Otolaryngol,* 36:71-78, 1942.

von Leden, H. V., and Isshiki, N.: An analysis of cough at the level of the larynx. *Arch Otolaryngol,* 81:616-625, 1965.

von Leden, H., and Moore, P.: Contact ulcer of the larynx. Experimental observations. *Arch Otolaryngol,* 72:746-752, 1960.

Voorhees, I. W.: Vocal fatigue in singers and speakers. *Trans Am Acad Ophthalmol Otolaryngol,* 19:340-348, 1914.

Wallner, L. J.: Smoker's larynx. *Laryngoscope,* 64:259-270, 1954.

Webb, W. W.: Papillomata of the larynx. *Laryngoscope,* 66:871-918, 1956.

Weiss, D. A.: The psychological relations to one's own voice. *Folia Phoniatr,* 7:209-217, 1955.

Weiss, D. A.: Functional treatment of paralysis of the recurrent nerve. *Internat Assoc Logopedics Phoniatr,* 14:380-383, 1968.

Weiss, D. A. and Beebe, H. H., (Eds.): *The Chewing Approach in Speech and Voice Therapy.* Basel, Switzerland, S. Karger, 1950.

Wendler, J., Igel, H., and Steindel, E.: Variations in vocal efficiency due to the menstruous cycle and how to influence them by ovulation inhibitors (Summary). *Internat Assoc Logopedics Phoniatr,* 14:247, 1968.

Werner-Kukuk, E., and von Leden, H.: Laryngeal trauma importance of objective laryngeal function tests. *Pract Otorhinolaryngol,* 31:166-173, 1969.

West, R., Ansberry, M., and Carr, A.: *The Rehabilitation of Speech,* 3rd ed. New York, Harper and Brothers, 1957.

West, R. A., Jr., Boggs, J. D., and Holinger, P. H.: Studies in tissue culture growth of laryngeal papilloma. *Acta Otolaryngol,* 48:14-15, 1957.

Weston, A., and Rousey, C.: The use of a tape recorder in clinical practice. *ASHA,* 12:551-552, 1970.

Wiksell, W. A.: An experimental analysis of respiration in relation to the intensity of vocal tones in speech. In Gray, G. W. (Ed.): *Studies in Experimental Phonetics, University Studies No. 27.* Baton Rouge, Louisiana St Univ Press, 1936, pp. 37-51.

Williamson, A. B.: Diagnosis and treatment of seventy-two cases of hoarse voice. *Q J Speech,* 31:189-202, 1945.

Williamson, A. B.: Symposium on adequacy of training of voice specialists. *Q J Speech,* 32:145-160, 1946.

Wilson, D. K.: Voice re-education of children with vocal nodules. *Laryngoscope,* 72:45-53, 1962a.

Wilson, D. K.: Voice reeducation of adolescents with vocal nodules. *Arch Otolaryngol,* 76:68-73, 1962b.

Wilson, D. K.: Voice re-education in benign laryngeal pathology. *Eye Ear Nose Throat Mon,* 45:76, 78-80, 1966.

Withers, B. T., and Dawson, M. H.: Psychological aspects . . . Treatment of vocal nodule cases. *Texas State J Med,* 56:43-46, 1960.

Wolberg, L. R.: The psychological management of individuals with speech and hearing problems. Part II/Conclusions. *J Commun Disord,* 1:75-84, 1967.

Wolski, W.: Hypernasality as the presenting symptom of myasthenia gravis. *J Speech Hear Disord,* 32:36-38, 1967.

Wolski, W., and Wiley, J.: Functional aphonia in a fourteen-year-old boy: A case report. *J Speech Hear Disord,* 30:71-75, 1965.

Yamashita, T.: Recurrent laryngeal nerve paralysis associated with endotracheal anesthesia. *J Oto-rhino-laryngol Soc Japan,* 68:1452-1459, 1965.

Yanagihara, N.: Acoustical studies on hoarseness. *Otorhinolaryngology Clinic* (Kyoto), 55:357-398, 1962.

Zaliouk, A.: The tactile approach in voice placement. *Folia Phoniatr,* 15:147-154, 1963.

Zilstorff, K.: Vocal disabilities of singers. *Proc R Soc Med,* 61:1147-1150, 1968.

APPENDICES

APPENDIX A

PATIENT REGISTRATION

(To Be Filled in Completely - Please Print)

OFFICE _____

DATE _____

PATIENT _____

FIRST   MIDDLE   LAST NAME   DATE OF BIRTH

RESPONSIBLE
PARTY _____ PHONE _____

(Full name of person responsible for payment of services, if other than Patient)
If Patient is a minor or another person is responsible, show following information regarding
responsible party. Otherwise, show information regarding Patient.

MARRIED ☐   DIVORCED ☐   WIDOW ☐   NAME OF HUSBAND OR WIFE _____

SINGLE ☐   SEPARATED ☐   WIDOWER ☐ _____

    FIRST NAME   MIDDLE NAME

RESIDENCE
ADDRESS _____

NO., STREET   CITY   ZIP CODE

EMPLOYER _____ OCCUPATION _____

EMPLOYER'S
ADDRESS _____

NO., STREET   CITY   PHONE

EMPLOYER OF
HUSBAND OR WIFE _____ OCCUPATION _____

EMPLOYER'S
ADDRESS _____

NO., STREET   CITY   PHONE

REFERRED
BY _____

NAME   ADDRESS   PHONE

M.D. _____ DIAGNOSIS _____

SURGERY _____

BASAL PITCH_____PND_____SINUSITUS_____

HOARSENESS_____COUGHING_____CLEARING THROAT_____

VOCAL FATIGUE_____VOCAL IMAGE_____MORNING VOICE_____

TONE FOCUS_____BREATH CONTROL_____

SMOKING_____ MENOPAUSE_____
　　　　　　YEARS　　　AMT. P/DAY

COLD_____ALLERGY_____ASTHMA_____OTHER_____

LENGTH OF TIME FOR PROBLEM_____

RECOGNIZE REPLAY_____REACTION_____

SESSIONS P/WK_____LENGTH OF SESSION_____COST_____

COST OF EVALUATION_____

COMMENTS:_____

APPENDIX B

NAME_____DATE_____

SENSORY SYMPTOMS   Eliminated

___1. Non-productive throat clearing
___2. Coughing
___3. Progressive vocal fatigue following brief or extended
       vocal usage
___4. Acute or chronic irritation or pain in or about larynx
       or pharynx
___5. Sternum pressure and/or pain
___6. Neck muscle cording
___7. Swelling of veins and/or arteries in the neck
___8. Throat stiffness
___9. Rapid vocal fatigue
___10. A feeling of a foreign substance or "lump" in throat
___11. Ear irritation or tickling or earache
___12. Repeated sore throats
___13. A tickling, tearing, soreness or burning sensation in
       the throat
___14. Scratchy or dry throat
___15. Tenderness of anterior and/or posterior strap muscles
___16. Rumble in chest
___17. Stinging sensation in soft palate
___18. A feeling that talking is an effort
___19. A choking feeling
___20. Tension and/or tightness in the throat
___21. Chronic toothache without apparent cause
___22. Back neck tension
___23. Headache
___24. Mucus formation
___25. Arytenoid tenderness
___26. Trachael pressure
___27. Anterior or posterior cervical pain
___28. Pain at base of tongue

AUDITORY SYMPTOMS

___1. Acute or chronic hoarseness
___2. Reduced vocal range
___3. Inability to talk at will and at length in variable
       situations
___4. Tone change from a clear voice to a breathy, raspy,
       squeaky, foggy, or rough voice
___5. Repeated loss of voice
___6. Laryngitis
___7. Voice breaks
___8. Voice skips
___9. Voice comes and goes during the day or over a period of
       months
___10. Clear voice in the morning with tired or foggy voice in the
       afternoon or evening
___11. Missed speech sounds

APPENDIX C

This is a voice questionnaire designed to assist you in determining the extent of your vocal abilities and disabilities.
Please help us in this review. There is no need to sign your
name unless you wish.

Male____   Female _____   Age_____

1. How would you rate your voice?
   Excellent___ Good___ Fair___ Poor___

2. How do you feel about the tone of your voice?
   Comfortable___ Uncomfortable___ Indifferent___

3. Have you experienced any of these symptoms during or after
   speaking?
   ___a. Tired voice
   ___b. Neck aches or pains
   ___c. Pressure at sternum
   ___d. Neck muscle cording
   ___e. Lump in throat
   ___f. Tickling, tearing, or burning sensation in throat
   ___g. Throat clearing
   ___h. Coughing
   ___i. Repeated sore throats
   ___j. Voice breaks and skips
   ___k. Loss of voice
   ___l. Pain at the back of the neck
   ___m. Dry throat
   ___n. Hoarseness

4. Have you experienced any vocal difficulty? Yes___ No___
   If so, has this affected you in any way? Yes___ No___
   Comment:

5. What type of voice do you like: Low pitch___ Medium pitch___
   High pitch___

6. Have you tried to use any of the following voices:
   ___a. A sexy voice
   ___b. A low-pitched voice
   ___c. A deep toned voice

7. Do your like your voice? Yes___ No___
   Would you want a different voice? Yes___ No___

8. Please specify the extent of voice training you have
   received for your speaking voice.
   a.___None
   b.___Course in public speaking
   c.___Other (Please specify)_____
   d.___What was your evaluation of the training?
       Excellent___ Good___ Fair___ Poor___

9. Would you want more or less training for your speaking voice?
   More___ Less___

10. How much do you smoke a day? _____packs.

THANK YOU FOR YOUR ASSISTANCE IN THIS STUDY

APPENDIX D

TEACHER QUESTIONNAIRE

Total Response = 179

	Female Nonsmokers	Male Nonsmokers	Female Smokers	Male Smokers
0-20	0	0	0	0
20-29	49	8	5	3
30-39	18	4	5	1
40-49	32	1	6	2
50-59	19	0	5	0
60-69	0	0	0	0
70+	0	0	0	0
Not given	14	3	2	2
TOTAL	132	16	23	8

1. How would you rate your voice?

Excellent	2	1	0	2
Good	70	7	9	3
Fair	53	8	9	2
Poor	3	0	2	0

2. How do you feel about the tone of your voice?

Comfortable	85	7	8	4
Uncomfortable	16	4	5	1
Indifferent	17	3	2	2

3. Have you experienced any of these symptoms during or after speaking?

Tired voice	42	7	11	4
Neck aches, pains	29	1	5	0
Pressure at sternum	3	0	0	0
Neck muscle cording	5	0	4	0
Lump in throat	17	0	3	2
Tickling, tearing, or burning in throat	22	4	9	1
Throat clearing	41	4	13	6
Coughing	14	4	6	5
Repeated sore throat	11	2	3	1
Voice breaks and skips	18	3	4	1
Loss of voice	11	2	4	2
Pain at back of neck	17	0	4	2
Dry throat	35	7	16	3
Hoarseness	34	5	11	2

Number of symptoms per patient:

0 Symptoms	29	3	2	0
1 Symptoms	30	4	1	1
2 Symptoms	30	1	2	1
3+ Symptoms	43	8	18	6

4. Have you experienced any vocal difficulty?

Yes	52	9	7	2
No	75	6	11	6

	Female Nonsmokers	Male Nonsmokers	Female Smokers	Male Smokers
If so, has this affected you in any way?				
Yes	46	4	5	2
No	3	2	2	0
5. What type of voice do you like?				
Low pitch	16	4	7	2
Medium pitch	107	11	14	6
High pitch	0	0	1	0
6. Have you tried to use any of the following voices?				
Sexy voice	6	2	7	1
Low-pitched voice	40	7	11	4
Deep-toned voice	7	6	5	2
7. Do you like your voice?				
Yes	94	9	13	7
No	31	6	3	1
Would you want a different voice?				
Yes	47	6	8	4
No	60	5	9	3
8. Please specify the extent of voice training you have received for your speaking voice.				
None	65	8	12	4
Public speaking	57	6	9	3
Other	15	3	2	4
What was your evaluation of the training?				
Excellent	6	0	1	0
Good	25	3	3	3
Fair	19	1	2	0
Poor	6	2	1	0
Would you want more or less training for your speaking voice?				
More	104	15	20	7
Less	0	0	0	0
How much do you smoke a day?				
0	132	16	0	0
0-½ pack	0	0	9	0
½-1 pack	0	0	6	2
1-2 pack	0	0	7	3
2-3	0	0	1	2
3+	0	0	0	0
Pipe	0	0	0	1

APPENDIX E

THEOLOGIANS

Total Response = 267

	Female Nonsmokers	Male Nonsmokers	Male Smokers
Under 21	1	0	0
21-30		18	0
31-40		40	7
41-50		51	2
51-60		31	9
61+	1	10	1
Not given		84	12
TOTAL	2	234	31

1. *How would you rate your voice?*

Excellent		41	6
Good		162	19
Fair	1	28	4
Poor	1	3	0

2. *How do you feel about the tone of your voice?*

Comfortable	1	209	27
Uncomfortable	1	14	1
Indifferent		9	2

3. *Have you experienced any of these symptoms during or after speaking?*

Tired voice	1	74	8
Neck aches or pains		7	0
Neck muscle cording		2	0
Lump in throat	1	13	0
Tickling, tearing, or burning sensation in throat	1	47	3
Throat clearing	2	74	6
Coughing		26	4
Repeated sore throats		8	0
Voice breaks and skips		21	0
Loss of voice	1	21	3
Pain at the back of the neck		7	0
Dry throat	2	48	6
Hoarseness	1	51	6

Number of symptoms per patient

0	0	68	12
1	0	65	8
2	0	40	5
3+	2	61	6

4. *Have you experienced any vocal difficulty?*

Yes	1	62	6
No	1	162	25

If so, has this affected you in any way?

Yes	1	25	1
No	1	37	5

	Female Nonsmokers	Male Nonsmokers	Male Smokers
5. *What type of voice do you like?*			
Low pitch	1	67	8
Medium pitch	1	165	20
High pitch	0	2	1
6. *Have you tried to use any of the following voices?*			
Sexy voice	1	18	1
Low-pitched voice	1	73	10
Deep-toned voice	0	58	7
None of the above voices	0	20	0
7. *Do you like your voice?*			
Yes	1	214	28
No	1	16	2
Would you want a different voice?			
Yes	1	36	5
No	1	167	23
8. *Please specify the extent of voice training you have received for your speaking voice.*			
None	0	32	3
Course in public speaking	2	175	26
Other	1	67	8
What was your evaluation of this training?			
Excellent	0	28	6
Good	1	92	10
Fair	1	37	4
Poor	0	1	0
9. *Would you want more or less training for your speaking voice?*			
More	2	182	19
Less	0	10	1
10. *How much do you smoke a day?*			
Under 1 pack			6
1-2 packs			8
2+ packs			1
Cigars			2
Pipes			14

APPENDIX F

GENERAL PUBLIC

Total Response = 432

	Female Nonsmokers	Male Nonsmokers	Female Smokers	Male Smokers
Under 21	3	2	0	1
21-30	41	25	5	6
31-40	40	34	4	4
41-50	57	33	14	3
51-60	46	21	6	1
61-70	5	4	1	0
70+	1	1	0	0
Not given	33	31	5	5
TOTAL	226	151	35	20

1. *How would you rate your voice?*

Excellent	1	10	1	1
Good	44	43	8	6
Fair	126	71	19	8
Poor	43	27	7	4

2. *How do you feel about the tone of your voice?*

Comfortable	64	42	7	7
Uncomfortable	112	80	20	7
Indifferent	32	26	7	5

3. *Have you experienced any of these symptoms during or after speaking?*

Tired voice	117	92	18	8
Neck aches or pains	37	19	5	0
Pressure at sternum	11	6	0	1
Neck muscle cording	24	15	4	1
Lump in throat	59	32	7	3
Tickling, tearing, or burning sensation	80	59	5	5
Throat clearing	109	100	23	9
Coughing	48	45	9	5
Repeated sore throat	48	29	2	3
Voice breaks and skips	68	49	12	6
Loss of voce	56	29	5	3
Pain at back of neck	25	10	5	1
Dry throat	96	85	14	11
Hoarseness	114	74	15	11
Number of symptoms per patient:				
0 symptoms	16	14	4	1
1 symptoms	27	15	4	4
2 symptoms	39	19	6	2
3+ symptoms	144	103	21	13

	Female Nonsmokers	Male Nonsmokers	Female Smokers	Male Smokers
4. *Have you experienced any vocal difficulty?*				
Yes	118	89	14	9
No	92	58	20	10
If so, has this affected you in any way?				
Yes	85	76	8	7
No	33	13	6	2
5. *What type of voice do you like?*				
Low pitch	56	53	8	7
Medium pitch	158	96	27	11
High pitch	3	0	0	0
6. *Have you tried to use any of the following voices?*				
Sexy voice	46	18	6	2
Low-pitched voice	106	62	16	5
Deep-toned voice	30	61	4	8
7. *Do you like your voice?*				
Yes	79	63	5	8
No	125	85	29	10
Would you want a different voice?				
Yes	141	103	24	13
No	60	37	6	5
8. *Please specify the extent of voice training you have received.*				
None	137	81	25	14
Course in public speaking	56	40	6	3
Other	27	26	4	3
What was your evaluation of this training?				
Excellent	6	10	1	1
Good	25	17	3	0
Fair	19	18	1	0
Poor	8	7	2	0
9. *Would you want more or less training for your speaking voice?*				
More	206	143	33	16
Less	1	3	0	1
10. *How much do you smoke a day?*				
Under 1 pack			19	5
1-2 packs			11	10
2+ packs			4	2
Cigars			1	1
Pipes			0	2

AUTHOR INDEX

A

Adler, S., 178-179, 315, 324
Alavi, S. M., 193, 326
Allen, K., 25, 322
Anderson, V. A., 16, 66-68, 97, 108, 123, 285, 315
Ansberry, M., 11, 16, 67, 205, 328
Arnold G. E., 5, 12, 164, 173, 187-188, 190, 198, 200-202, 315, 324
Aronson, A. E., 167-169, 173, 315
Ash, J. E., 12, 15, 316

B

Baker, D. C., 5, 12, 192, 316
Bangs, J. L., 168, 316
Barbara, D. A., 322
Baron, S. H., 27, 316
Barton, R. T., 168, 316
Bauer, H., 29, 316
Baynes, R., 153, 316
Beebe, H. H., 67, 69, 328
Bergström, J., 27, 316
Bicknell, J. M., 173, 316
Bjork, H., 192, 316
Bloch, E. L., 36, 316
Bloch, P., 35, 65, 173, 316
Boedts, D., 198, 316
Boggs, J. D., 192, 328
Boland, J. L., 17, 23, 317
Bonneville, J., 29, 321
Boone, D. R., 85, 168, 317, 319
Brewer, D. W., 14, 24, 317
Briess, F. B., 14, 24, 197, 317
Brodnitz, F. S., 11-12, 18, 25, 29, 34, 56, 66, 68, 72, 108, 125, 143, 146, 167, 169, 179, 194, 197, 274-275, 282-283, 285, 317
Brown, B. S., 198, 327
Brown, J. R., 315
Brumlik, J., 173, 326

Bryant, L. R., 193, 326
Bryngelson, B., 163, 317
Byrne, D., 326

C

Calvet, J., 29, 317
Canter, G. J., 202, 317
Carr, A., 11, 16, 67, 205, 328
Carrell, J., 34, 208, 317
Cavanaugh, J. A., 14, 317
Chiong, A. T., 271-272, 320
Clerf, L. H., 8, 13, 318
Coates, H. M., 323
Coll, J., 29, 317
Cooper, M., 12, 15, 17-18, 20-21, 23, 36-37, 41, 56, 68-69, 75, 126-127, 153, 158-159, 171, 189-190, 194, 198, 274, 318-319, 326
Corbetta, L., 27, 319
Cornut, C., 17, 319
Cornut, G., 17, 50, 198, 273, 319
Cracovaner, A. J., 15, 197, 319
Craik, J. E., 12, 323
Cunning, D. S., 272, 319
Curry, E. T., 153, 319

D

Damste, P. H., 29, 319
Darley, F. L., 143-144, 319
Davis, D. S., 85, 319
Dawson, M. H., 15, 329
Dekelboum, A., 192, 320
Delaini, A., 202
Dellon, A. L., 22, 322
Denney, R., 33, 326
Devine, K. D., 12, 192, 324-325
Diehl, C., 179, 320
Dieleman, F., 29, 327
Doehler, M., 211, 320
Douglas, T. E., 62, 320
Dreher, J. J., 178, 324

343

SUBJECT INDEX

A

Accents, 26
Acceptability of voice problem and rehabilitation, 131
Adenoidectomy, 22, 180
Adolescent dysphonias, 156-157 (*see also* Children)
Aesthetic voice, 41-42, 123-125
Age and dysphonias, 153-158
Aggravated voice, 5, 17
Air conditioning, 26
Airplane travel, 9
Alcohol, 15, 197
Allergies, 22, 26, 28
Amytrophic lateral sclerosis, 5, 204
Anabolic steroids, 29
Anatomical abnormalities, 22
Anger, 33
Ankylosis of cricoarytenoid joint, 28
Antibiotics, 55, 58-59
Anxieties, 10
Aphonia defined, 166
Arteries, swelling of, 7
Articulation problems, 26
Artistic voice, 125-126
  defined, 125
  efficient voice compared, 125
  pitch and, 126
Arytenoid edema, 27
Arytenoid tenderness, 7
Associate therapy, 55, 71, 105-108, 120, 132, 157
  children, 106-107
  benefits from, 108
  defined, 105
  falsetto voice, 160
  function of, 107
  hindering effect of, 107
  nasality, 183
  need for, 106
Audibility, 25

Auditory symptoms of dysphonia, 6-8, 10-11, 277-278
Authoritarian voice, 44, 49-50
Automation carry-over technique, 96-97
Automobile accidents, medicolegal aspects of voice disorders from, 272-273

B

Back neck tension, 7
Ball games, 9
Basal pitch, 18-24, 39, 45-50, 77, 87 (*see also specific voice disorders*)
  authoritarian voice, 49-50
  confidential voice, 45
  defined, 18
  falsetto voice, 160-161
  fluctuation in, 18-19
  intimate voice, 45
  low-pitched vocal image voice, 20
  morning voice, 20-21
  post-sleep voice, 20-21
  sexy voice, 48
  telephone voice, 47
  vocal misuse and, 18-21
Bed rest, 55, 62
Bedroom voice, 44, 48-49
Belch sound, method of producing, 211
Benign growths and lesions, 13-14, 197
  surgery, 55-58
Bibliography, 315-329
Bibliotherapy, 55, 71, 108, 120, 131-132
Bodily fatigue, 26, 32
Body image, 38
Bowed vocal folds, 5-6, 184-186
  myasthenia laryngis distinguished, 184-185
  paralytic dysphonia distinguished, 184-185
  vocal rehabilitation, 184-186

347

U

"Um-hum" method, 74-77, 80-81, 169
Upper chest breathing, 24-25, 42-43, 89
Upper respiratory infection, 26, 30-32, 59, 136, 166, 173

V

Vacations, 55, 62
Vaporizers, 55, 61
Veins, swelling of, 7
Ventricular phonation, 5-6, 164-165, 224-225 (Charts)
 defined, 164
 prognosis, 165
 self-induced, 164
 vocal misuse, 164
 vocal rehabilitation, 165
  results of, 165, 224-225 (Charts), 275-282, 286-289 (Charts)
  results of follow-up, 282-284, 311-313 (Charts)
Virus infection, 191-192
Visual symptoms of dysphonia, 6-8, 10-11, 277-278
Vocal abuse, 153 (see also specific topics and specific voice disorders)
 acute, 9
 alleviation of, 9
 auditory symptoms, 10-11
 causes of, 11
 chronic, 9-10
 constitutional factors, 26-32
 defined, 8
 elimination of, 9
 environmental factors, 26-32
 excessive use of voice distinguished, 15-16
 functional misphonia, 12
 habitual, 10
 lesions and growths, 12-15
 malignancies, 14-15
 maltreatment, 9
 neurological involvement, 12
 overuse of voice distinguished, 15-16
 patient's awareness of, 125
 physical contributory factors to, 26-32

premalignancies, 12-14, 196
 psychological contributory factors to, 32-52
 recurrence of growths, 56-57
 results of, 12-15
 sensory symptoms, 10-11
 stages of, 10-11
 visual symptoms, 10-11
 vocal misuse following, 10
Vocal awareness, 137
Vocal catharsis, 103
Vocal concepts, misguided, 11
Vocal cues, 103-104
Vocal fatigue, 7, 16
Vocal folds
 carcinoma, 12-14, 206
 edema, 8, 13
 growths and lesions, 5-6, 12-15, 22-23, 157
  differential diagnosis, 271-272
 impairment of, 22
 inflammation, 8, 13, 22-23, 27-28
 irritation, 13, 27-28
 mistreatment of, 8
 paralysis of (see Paralytic dysphonia)
 premalignant lesions, 12-14
 redness, 8
 thickening, 13
Vocal fry, 19
 classification of, 19
 defined, 19
Vocal hygiene, 127-128, 136, 206-207
 adolescent dysphonias, 156
 children, 155-156
 singers, 127
Vocal image, 9, 11, 24, 36-44, 109 (see also specific voice disorders)
 absence of, 38-39
 alteration of, 99-100
 body image, influence of, 38
 breath support image, 36-37, 42-43
 child, 52
 defined, 36
 esophageal voice patients, 209, 215-218
 formation of, factors contributing to, 37-39
 influences upon, 37-39

Voice training and inadequacies and
    needs, 284-286
Voice types, 44-50 *(see also specific
    type)*
  conscious manipulation, 44-45
  rehabilitation requirements, 50
  unconscious acquisition, 44-45
Volume, 5, 8-9, 66 *(see also specific
    voice disorders)*
  excessive, 24, 88-89
  inadequate, 24, 87
  modern therapy methods, 71, 87-90

  carry-over of, 92
  need for, 122-123
  vocal misuse and, 23-24
  voice types and, 45-50
Volume image, 36, 42

W

Whispering, 60

Y

Yelling, 24 (*see also* Screaming; Shout-
    ing)